LIVE
YOUNG
FOREVER

12 Steps to Optimum
Health, Fitness & Longevity

"Longevity is a blessing and by leading a healthy lifestyle and nourishing ourselves both physically and spiritually, we can live a life of great fulfillment."

Hazel McCallion, C.M.,
Runner-up, World Mayor

For Men and Women

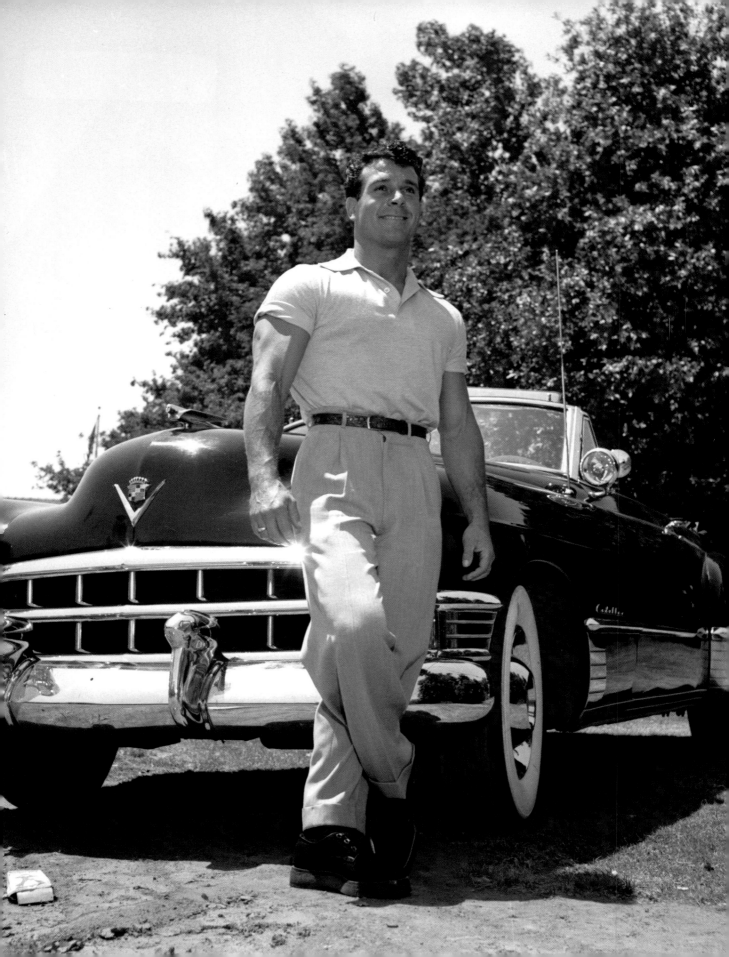

JACK LALANNE

LIVE
YOUNG
FOREVER

12 Steps to Optimum
Health, Fitness & Longevity

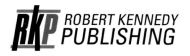

RKP ROBERT KENNEDY PUBLISHING

Published by Robert Kennedy Publishing
400 Matheson Blvd. West
Mississauga, ON
L5R 3M1 Canada
Visit us at **www.shopRKpubs.com** and
www.LiveYoungWithJackLalanne.com

Senior Production Editor: Wendy Morley
Online and Associate Editor: Vinita Persaud
Junior Production Editor: Cali Hoffman
Editorial Assistant: Lili Pusic
Art Director: Gabriella Caruso Marques
Assistant Art Director: Jessica Pensabene
Editorial Designer: Brian Ross

Library and Archives Canada Cataloguing in Publication

LaLanne, Jack, 1914-
    Live young forever / Jack LaLanne.

ISBN 978-1-55210-064-6

    1. Middle-aged persons--Health and hygiene. 2. Middle-aged
persons--Nutrition. 3. Physical fitness for middle-aged persons.
I. Title.

RA777.5.L35 2009   613'.0434   C2009-902013-0

10 9 8 7 6 5 4 3 2 1

Distributed in Canada by
NBN (National Book Network)
67 Mowat Avenue, Suite 241
Toronto, ON
M6K 3E3

Distributed in USA by
NBN (National Book Network)
15200 NBN Way
Blue Ridge Summit, PA
17214

Printed in Canada

IMPORTANT

The information in this book reflects the authors' experiences and opinions and is not intended to replace medical advice.

Before beginning this or any nutritional or exercise regimen, consult your physician to be sure it is appropriate for you. Ask for a physical stress test.

SPECIAL THANKS

I have so many people in my life I would like to thank from the bottom of my athletic heart. First on the list is my wife, Elaine, who has stood behind me and encouraged me for over 50 years. She is the power behind my muscles. I would also like to thank my publisher, Robert Kennedy, for his excitement and encouragement in my doing this book, along with senior editor Wendy Morley, for her dedication and countless hours coordinating this project. On my end, kudos to my son, Danny, my office assistants, Karleyne Binford, Colleen Amick and Claire Ipekjian, who were instrumental in helping research the facts and inputting my comments into the computer, since my computer skills are limited and my typewriter broke back in 1978. Dr. Gale Rudolph, my nutritionist and collaborator of over 40 years, also helped review the nutritional aspects of the book. My other family members are also important to me so I would like to acknowledge my daughter, Dr. Yvonne LaLanne, DC, her husband, Dr. Mark Rubenstein, MD, and my son Jon Allen and his wife Lora LaLanne.

The following people contributed moral support, humor and just plain friendship:

Rusty Duclos

Carol & Dan Grant

Ariel Hankin

Rick Hersh

Ed Labowitz, Esq.

Dr. Anthony Lauro, DC

Josef & Jamie Lavi

Keith & Anjali Merchandani

Joon & Jina Oh

Evelyn Reichel

Dr. Roger Russo, DC

Jeff Vicars

Barry Zegel & crew at CBS TVC

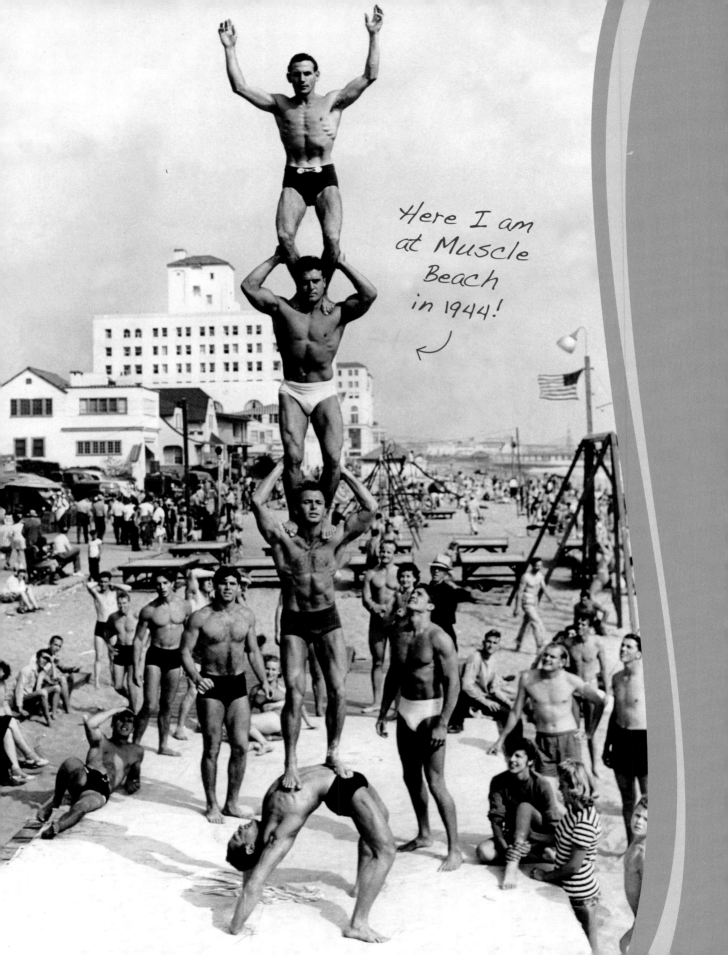

Here I am at Muscle Beach in 1944!

CONTENTS

		Foreword by Robert Kennedy	8
		Introduction	12
One	■	Early Craziness	16
Two	■	My Plan for You	28
Three	■	Far from Perfect	40
Four	■	Step 1: Motivation	50
Five	■	Step 2: Step Away from Killer Habits	60
Six	■	Step 3: Personal Care	74
Seven	■	Step 4: Eating Clean	88
Eight	■	Step 5: Maintain Perfect Posture	108
Nine	■	Step 6: Stay Well Hydrated	116
Ten	■	Step 7: Stretching	124
Eleven	■	Step 8: Find Some Energy	138
Twelve	■	Step 9: Be in a Solid Relationship	148
Thirteen	■	Step 10: Work Out	154
Fourteen	■	Step 11: Never Retire	198
Fifteen	■	Step 12: Consume Plenty of Fruits and Vegetables	204
Sixteen	■	My Wish for You	272
		Jack LaLanne Achievement Timeline	276
		Credits	284
		Index	285

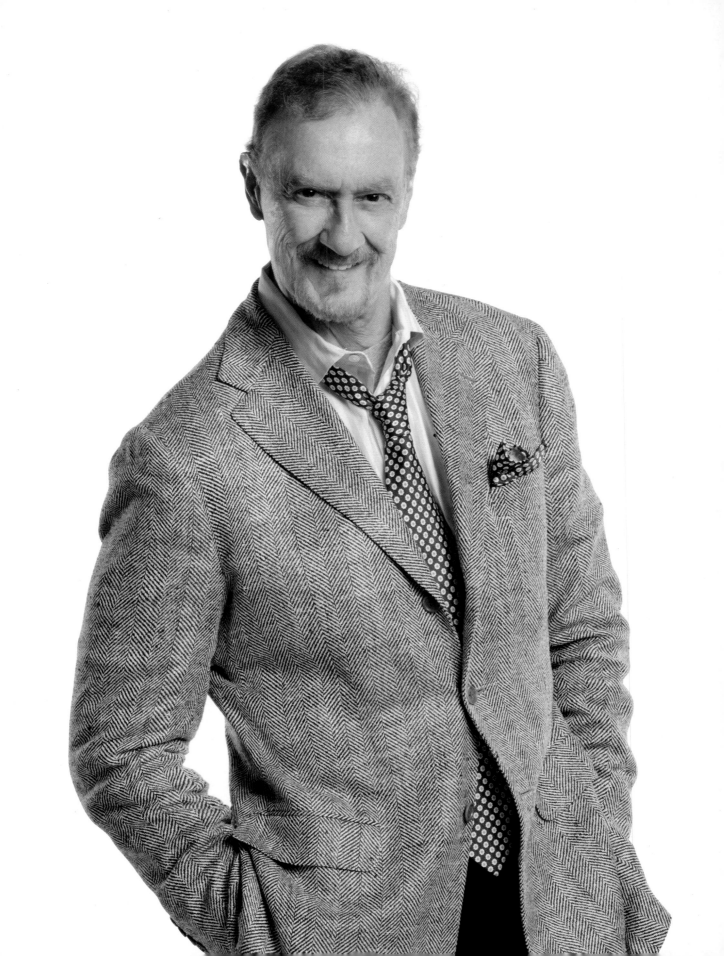

FOREWORD

BY ROBERT KENNEDY

Back in 1936 Jack LaLanne, at 21 years of age, opened North America's first modern gym. It was on the third floor of an old office building in Oakland, California. He paid $45 a month for rent. He was ridiculed for his concept of actually charging people to exercise, but the place was packed with members.

As the years went by his basic approach to physical fitness and nutrition was established as scientifically sound. Jack developed the first models of exercise equipment, and these are standard in gyms today. He came up with the first leg extension machine, the first pulley machines using cables and the first weight selectors. He was the first to have women work out with weights – a radical idea. He also encouraged the disabled and elderly to exercise for health, a bizarre concept at the time.

Today at 95 years of age, Jack is extremely flexible and has a will and mind as sharp as a tack. His wife Elaine, herself active, fit and svelte at 84, says she has known Jack for 60 years and has never known him to be sick.

Jack, from whom the term "jumping jacks" and the description of a muscular person as "jacked" are both derived, is well known for his birthday feats. At age 70 the guy towed 70 boats carrying 70 people across the Long Beach Harbor, with both arms and feet shackled. This prompted the question by writer Diane Cyr: If men are from Mars and women are from Venus, what planet did Jack LaLanne come from? Jack insists he's from planet Earth, adding: "I was the worst, most sickly kid of all — 30 pounds underweight. The girls used to beat me up. Actually, I was a mean kid early on because I had no self-esteem." What saved him as a teenager is what maintains him now: exercise, diet and positive thinking. "There is no fountain of youth," says Jack. "What you put in your body is what you get out of it. You wouldn't feed your dog a coffee and a doughnut for breakfast followed by a cigarette. You'd kill the damn dog!"

Jack has written *Live Young Forever* because he genuinely believes in his way of life (he personally gets up at five in the morning to exercise). He understands that for some, working out can be difficult at first, but once you get it you totally get it. Then you fully grasp that the benefits outweigh the tribulations involved with eating clean all the time and keeping to a routine of formal exercise.

"The emphasis is in YOU," says Jack. He believes in the higher power, the Creator ("The Good Book says we are fearfully and wonderfully made — believe it!"). But Jack also believes we have to keep our end of the mortal bargain. "God gives us the power to act for ourselves, but let me tell you something. At five in the morning I've never heard this," he says, mimicking a knock on the door. "Hello Jack, this is Jesus. I'll work out for you today."

Jack LaLanne is tough on himself. When it comes to choosing between a down-filled pillow and the cold chin-up bar, there's no question. Give Jack LaLanne half a chance and he will talk about the magic of exercise and good nutrition for hours. Yet strangely he seldom mentions the names of various celebrities he has helped to find the true fitness formula. The list includes numerous presidents and prime ministers, movie stars, politicians and industry big wigs, but it's unlikely you'll hear that from Jack.

Also I should mention that as serious as Jack is about living a healthy lifestyle, he is no prude. He has an enormous, sometimes slightly raunchy sense of humor. He is very much part of this world and enjoys a good laugh. Life for him is sheer joy. At one of his talks some 30 years ago, the previous speaker was given a roof-lifting standing ovation. As Jack came to the podium, he looked a little shocked and feigned a degree of dismay. "Wow!" he said, "I feel a little like Elizabeth Taylor's eighth husband. I know what to do, but how do I make it interesting?"

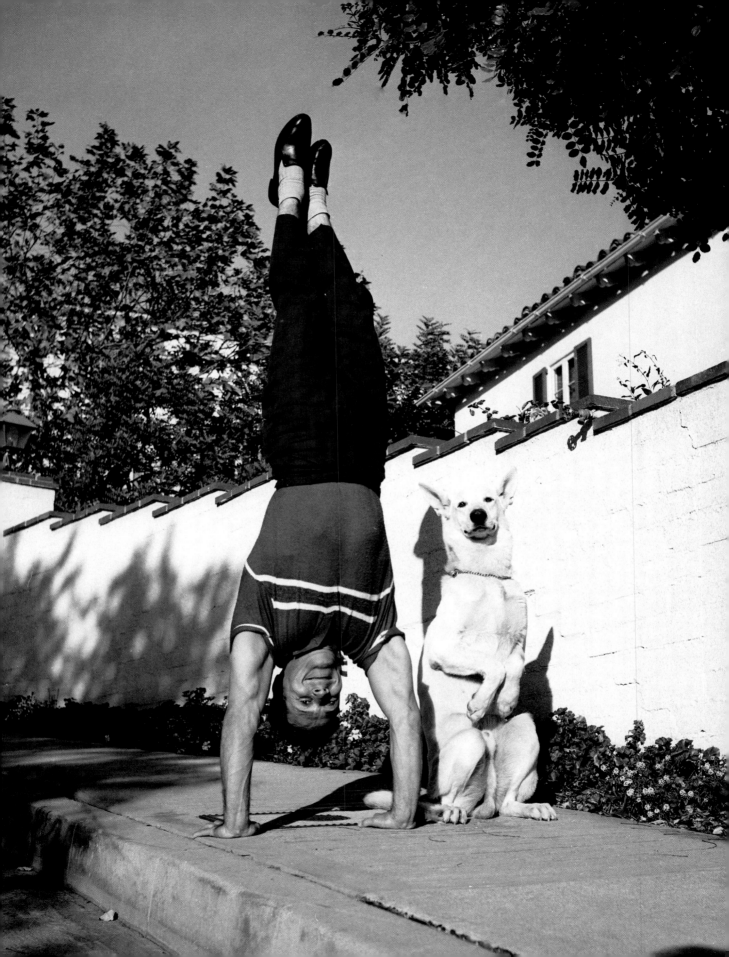

INTRODUCTION

BY JACK LALANNE

Here I am now at 95 years of age. I've just come back from a fantastic dinner overlooking the Pacific Ocean with my beautiful wife Elaine. We enjoyed a bowl of vegetable soup, broiled fish, a salad of 10 different raw vegetables and some fresh fruit for dessert. For our upcoming anniversary, we toasted each other with a glass of red wine. Elaine and I often meet old and new friends when eating out. The most common question I am asked is: "Jack, how do you do it? How do you keep up the pace of daily workouts and eating only the healthiest of foods? Don't you ever get tempted to fall off the wagon?" My answer to them is: "You bet I do! But I don't do it!" I have a serious sweet tooth which I satisfy by eating fresh fruit. As far as exercise is concerned, it's pretty tough sometimes leaving a warm bed and a hot woman at five in the morning to go into a cold gym, but I do it because it's my chosen way of life and I like the results.

I don't tell others to follow me through my extensive two-hour morning weight-training routine and swim, but I do feel it is extremely important that you do some exercise at least three or four days a week. The foods you eat are also important. They should be only the most nutritious foods, and as I often say, "If man makes it, don't eat it!" I do my best to avoid anything in a can or a box. When you eat healthy and exercise, your whole life can change for the better. In other words, you become A NEW YOU!

I don't care how old you are. It doesn't matter. Whether you are a man or woman, tall or short, fat or thin, young or not so young, my advice applies to you. It is advice that comes from the heart. Until now millions of people have sought in vain for the miraculous fountain of youth to wash away the misery of obesity or the infirmities of old age. They seek to step forward to new health and energy, wishing to shed unwanted weight and to further shape and tone the muscles of the body. This book will help you find real answers. I live my life as an example, to show people I practice what I preach. The response from the public has been overwhelmingly positive for the last 75 years.

Why did I write this book? Do I need the money? Do I even want the money? No way!

At age 95, my reason for writing this book is to get the health and fitness word out to the world one more time. I realize the combination of exercise and good nutrition is better understood than ever before, but sadly millions of us are not following a sensible path to ensure lifelong health and fitness.

For some of us the aging process seems to take hold in our teens. We have only to look at our schoolchildren to see the heavy waistlines and the pathetic state of fitness levels caused by lazy lifestyles and modern technology – TVs, computers, Facebook, Twitter, text messaging, video games and more, all of which encourage physical inactivity.

The next time you go to the movies take a look around. You see men, women and children loaded up with sugary soft drinks, popcorn slathered with golden topping and chocolate bars even if they've just finished dinner! How about the habit of grabbing a quick meal at some fast-food establishment? Many North Americans habitually eat and drink junk foods through take-out or fast-food restaurants. Always remember this: What you eat today will be walking and talking tomorrow. Never doubt it!

Today you may be relatively young but now is the time to outwit old age. With your new health, strength and fitness level, your body will thank you for your efforts. Believe me, once you adopt the simple principles of life mentioned in this book, you will never look back. You will feel energetic and fit. Life will have a new joy. You will shed unwanted pounds and look like a million dollars. Make that two million dollars! I don't want to end this introduction on a sour note, but one day I will be gone. My sincere wish is that you follow my advice to live as long and healthy a life as I have. Keep this book handy for when you feel like giving up. My hopes and aspirations are for your personal health, strength, fitness and longevity for all your days. I have your highest achievements in mind. If you know me, you may have read or heard me say, time and time again, **"Anything in life is possible and YOU make it happen"**!

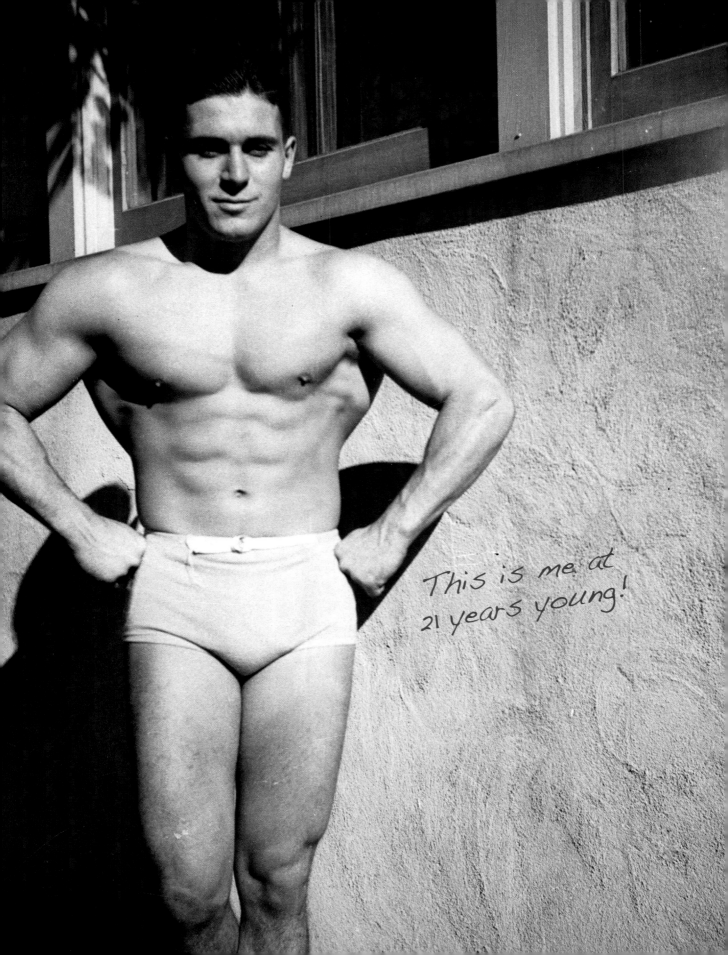

This is me at 21 years young!

CHAPTER ONE

Early
Craziness

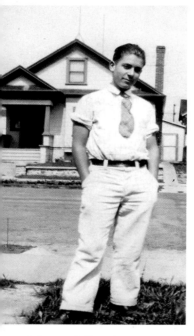

Myself at age 15.

It took me a while, but I figured a few things out. Hey! As I write this ... I'm above ground, happy as anyone on this crazy mud ball we call Earth and loving every minute of life to the fullest. It wasn't always that way. As a kid I was addicted to sugar and junk food and this would contribute to my having crazy moods.

My personal adventure began when I was three years old. I am told that I was a very hyper kid. I loved sweet things, so if I became rambunctious, to appease me, my mother would take a cloth with sugar and dip it in water and I would suck on it. Sugar was my reward for everything. My health got so bad doctors recommended my parents take me to a more temperate climate. Hence, we moved to the hot dry flats of the Bakersfield area, where my grandfather had a sheep ranch in Greenfield. The ranch should have been an ideal place for the development of health and strength, because all the components were there; sun, fresh air, spring water, fruits and vegetables, but something was very wrong.

Our pumpkins and pears won blue ribbons at the County Fair. Our livestock were fed only the best fodder. I remember that a lot of money was spent on feeding the sheep the best food to bring the best prices for our stock. While all this was going on our entire family gave absolutely no thought whatsoever to their own nutritional needs. We simply ate and drank what tasted good. There were no blue ribbons for the LaLannes. The truth is we lived for the farm. All attention was for the ranch creatures. My mother, a tiny woman to begin with, paid less attention to her own state of health than she would to a sick ewe. We lived for our work rather than by it. Neighboring farms were no different. The

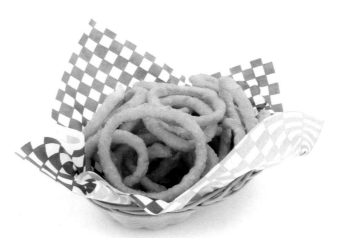

Hearing the message somehow doesn't translate to *getting* the message.

farm hands were eating packaged foods rather than fresh fruits, eggs, poultry and vegetables.

Looking back those 80-plus years today, I can see clearly what was happening. We lived by the barter system. We produced the best corn, fruit, eggs and vegetables in the area. And what did we do with it? We trucked it into town and traded it for white bread, pastries, candies, packaged foods and dessert preparations that looked tempting in the ads of the time. We traded away our birthright of health, energy and body shape. Our degree of ignorance was sad.

It was there, as a boy, that I developed a huge hunger and a liking for candy and soft drinks. No one had taught me to eat correctly because no one at our ranch knew how, or cared. No one thought nutrition was important. The vegetables that we did eat were drastically overcooked, tasteless and soggy. (God bless you Mom. You just didn't know.) I ended up hating vegetables, but I loved – yes loved – chocolate bars, pie, cake and ice cream. They were great! And not for a second did I consider that these "foods" were anything but healthy nutrition.

We have the same situation today. Even more so. We live in a land of plenty yet we continue to eat the most atrocious foods imaginable. And worse, we encourage our children to do the same. Fast-food restaurants are teeming with both adults and kids who just don't know the damage they are doing to themselves. But they should know. After all, magazines, newspapers, Internet sites and TV all go on about the singular message for health, fitness and longevity. That message? It's the importance of eating wholesome non-manufactured foods and exercising regularly. But *hearing* the message somehow doesn't translate to *getting* the message.

My own youth from ages 10 to 14 was miserable. I never smiled. My teeth were discolored; I was a real junk-food junkie. I became a psychological eater. One time I even sneaked a dollar from my mother's purse to buy ice cream and candy. I would trade my lunch sandwiches any day for sugar donuts. As a result I developed uncontrollable rages. My brother and I were always fighting. He was six years older and I wanted to be like him. He would tell me "You can't do that, kid." I was so skinny and scrawny that even the girls use to beat me up. I would get terrible headaches sometimes so bad that I would hit my head against the wall.

Our school in Greenfield was a one room schoolhouse with eight grades. I was a trouble maker and would get into a fight almost every day. Not only would the teacher give me a beating but when I got home I got another beating from my uncle because I screwed up in school.

I became a psychological eater.

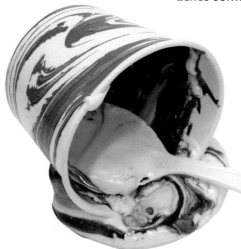

I was prone to fevers and they came frequently. Once when I was about 13 I became seriously ill and out of my head with a temperature of 104 for about 14 days. I was a raving maniac and tried to shoot my brother with my uncle's 22 shotgun. Another time I tried to set the house on fire. By the end of the 14th day, the doctors said I probably wouldn't live through the night. But my mother's aunt had talked my mother into becoming a Seventh Day Adventist and she got all the members of her church together for an all-night prayer session for me. Mom got on her knees and said "Dear God, if you will spare Jack's life I will never eat meat again." (Seventh Day Adventists are vegetarians.) By morning, whether miraculously or by coincidence, my fever broke. The doctors couldn't believe it. From then on, my mother never had a piece of meat and lived to be 94.

But more was to come. A swelling developed behind my left ear. One day a friend accidentally hit it with a basketball. That caused me to scream at the top of my lungs. My temperature was 104 by the time the doctor got to me. They operated immediately on an abscess which, had it not been attended to without further delay, would have traveled and infected my brain. My body was hitting rock bottom. I wore glasses, had a back brace to support my weak shoulders, and used arch supports in my shoes. Because I was still a sugarholic and kept up my daily consumption of colas, chocolate and candies, I continued to suffer from depression and loneliness. Life was a drag. As I write this, even 80 years later, I am reliving those dreadful years. I still feel the pain.

About this same time when I was 13, my grandfather passed away. Not only did he pass away, but just before the Big Depres-

My body was hitting rock bottom.

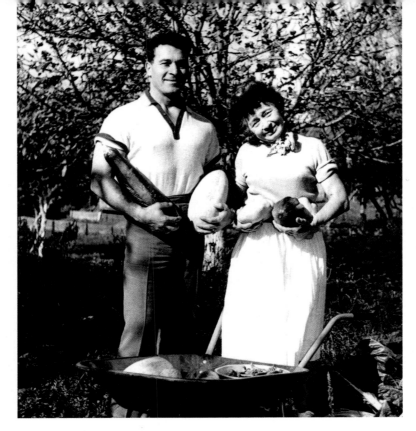

My mother and me. She lived to be 94!

sion hit, our sheep, that were eating better than we were, contracted hoof-and-mouth disease. They all died from tainted feed just before they were to be sold. We couldn't pay our bills and the Bank of Italy foreclosed on the ranch. My mother, father, brother, uncle and I went back to the bay area, to Berkeley, California. My father went to work for the telephone company, where he had worked before. I was still a very sick kid; in fact I had to drop out of school I was so sick and then a simple event occurred that totally changed my life.

A sympathetic neighbor, aware of my sickly disposition, got tickets for my mother and me to attend a Paul Bragg seminar at the Women's City Club in Oakland. We arrived a little late and the place was packed. I was wearing glasses at the time and my face was a mass of pimples and boils. I was embarrassed and secretly pleased that there were no seats. We started to leave. Then, the lecturer Paul Bragg called out, "Lady with the little boy.

We don't turn anyone away! Ushers bring up two seats and put them onstage." Two folding chairs were placed onstage and my mother and I sat in front of all these people for the entire seminar. It was the most embarrassing moment of my life, but gradually I forgot my position and became engrossed in what Mr. Bragg had to say: "My dear friends, it matters not what your age is; it matters not what your present physical condition is. If you obey nature's laws, you can be born again." My mouth was open wide as I listened to this man talking about building the body, eating correctly and exercising. Everything he said made sense. I was instantly converted to the health-and-fitness lifestyle. Bragg said I could be born again. That is exactly what I wanted. I had a desire to be an athlete. I wanted better grades in school. I wanted to be popular with girls.

Paul Bragg seemed like a prophet. He appeared to be speaking directly to me. He described my woes perfectly, and he offered hope. I could have the whole new life he promised – I just had to feed myself properly and exercise correctly. He was offering a brand new, exciting existence that would lift me out of my anguish. I bought every word, and added all the fervor of youth. I was off on the biggest adventure of my life. That night I became a vegetarian. I swore off all junk food. I determined that it was indeed the first night of my real, born-again life.

Today I can see that I was too radical, the self-directed kind. I had no scientific training for what I was doing. I simply followed the various ideas that seemed to make sense at the time. I decided then to learn everything possible about health and nutrition, reading everything from *Gray's Anatomy* to muscle-building magazines

I was off on the biggest adventure of my life!

to medical journals. I was getting educated. Still in my teens, I was searching; I was on a quest.

Although I felt infinitely better than I had in the past, eventually I decided I needed some animal protein because I felt tired, sleepy and frequently had gas pains. My diet lacked amino acids. I discovered the protein value in egg whites and later fish. I felt better immediately. That's not to say I disagree with people who choose vegetarianism. It's just that when I became active in sports and weight training I found that some animal protein, especially fish, helps decrease my recuperation time after workouts and seemed to give me more stamina.

In these teen years I was crazy, eager to try anything. A man came to town. He had amazing skin and hair. Even his fingernails were perfect. He said he had a surefire formula: soak grapefruit rinds all night, boil them in the morning and drink the juice. I tried his recipe and lo and behold my hair, skin and nails looked 100 percent better. When I later learned that I could get the same results from eating oranges I took the nightly grapefruit rinds off the stove.

I went overboard a different way another time I began experimenting with weightlifting with heavy cement blocks in my backyard. After lifting those heavy blocks every day for hours, I hurt my back so bad I couldn't train anymore. Having tried to find a cure without success, I learned of a doctor in Salt Lake City who swore by fresh vegetables juices. "They are full of potent minerals," he argued, stating that such juices could heal muscular injuries. It made sense to me, so I tried it — I mixed celery and carrot juice together and drank two quarts a day. This seemed to

> **In my teen years I was crazy, eager to try anything.**

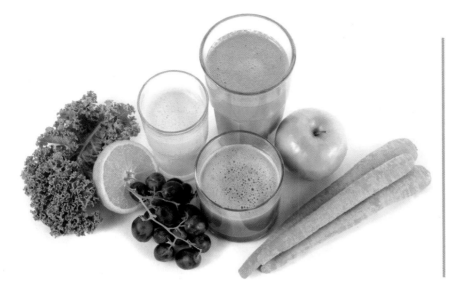

help my back problem but the excessive amount of carrot juice turned my skin orange. I found later I could have gotten by with half a pint of juice and had the same result. Gradually I learned my lesson about moderation. Just because one apple is good for you, it doesn't mean that 80 apples will do 80 times as much good. Nutrition doesn't work that way!

At age 15 I joined the Berkeley YMCA and got on their wrestling team. One day I saw these guys using weights. I asked if I could use them too. They said no. I said: "If I wrestle you guys and pin you will you let me use them?" They laughed, I pinned them and that was the beginning of my life-long career.

Soon after I went to the foundry, bought weights and started a gym in my backyard in Berkeley. Before long I had police officers and firemen working out with me and was able to collect enough money to buy more weights and gain more students.

My senior year in high school I really started to enjoy life. I played quarterback on the varsity football team, wrestled for the YMCA, and took up shot put, high jump, basketball, and pole vault for the "B" teams. After my earlier unhappiness I felt like an all-American boy, bursting with energy, doing well in my studies, enjoying female company for the first time and perhaps becoming a little bit of a showoff to overcome my timidity. Even today in front of crowds of fans I'm self-conscious until I feel that my audience is with me. The only time I'm completely without shyness is when I'm 100 percent into actively helping someone else better their lives.

Some years after graduating I read about a tribe in Africa whose members were taller and healthier than neighboring tribes. These people drank quantities of blood from their herds of cattle. The warriors drank it straight while the women mixed it with goat's milk. It all made sense. The taste of good meat is in the juice, with enzymes intact. I was convinced that by drinking blood not only would I get stronger, but my height too would increase. "Got to get me some of that," I said. So off I went to the local slaughterhouse in Oakland. I was greeted with cynicism, laughter, ridicule and disdain from the workers when I turned up every morning for my quart of blood. "Hey guys, Jack's here! Come and watch him drink his breakfast!" I created a lot of amusement and the most common remark was, "Better you than me, Jack." "Is it working, Jack? You don't seem to be growing." "Jack, you gotta be a crazy guy. How could you drink that stuff?"

I drank blood every day for weeks, until that is, one fateful day when I got a blood clot stuck in my throat. That was the end of my blood-drinking nutrition program. No more visits to the slaughterhouse. Today I wince at the very thought of drinking blood. I can't imagine how I even did it.

I was greeted with cynacism, laughter, ridicule and distain.

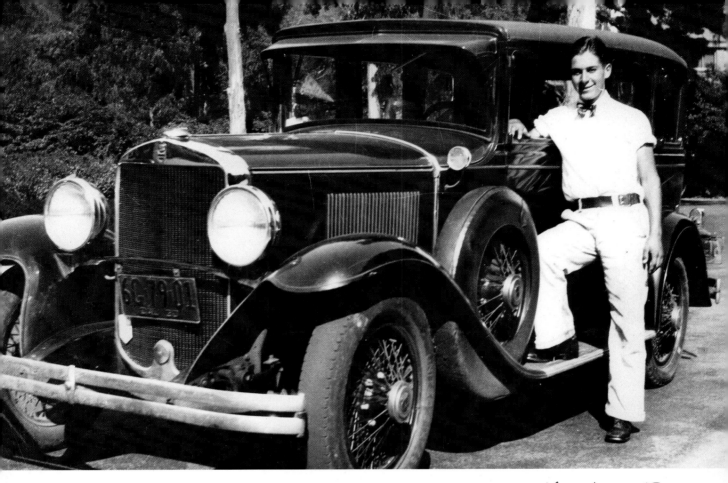

Me at age 18.

One day when I had written my first book back in 1960 I was at a Hollywood party when Hedda Hopper, the famous gossip columnist, approached me. "Are you going to deliver a copy of your book together with a quart of blood to all your friends, Jack?" "No, Hedda," I replied. "The blood thing was a little radical and it didn't seem to be working. If anything now, I would deliver a whole cow."

I went a little overboard. In my quest for health and happiness, I decided to normalize my eating habits. My school lunch now contained whole-wheat sandwiches, apples and oranges. I was getting all my protein from nuts, legumes and grains. But in truth, I didn't mind at all that my classmates began calling me "Health Nut" instead of their former taunt: "Bellyacher." Life was getting better every day.

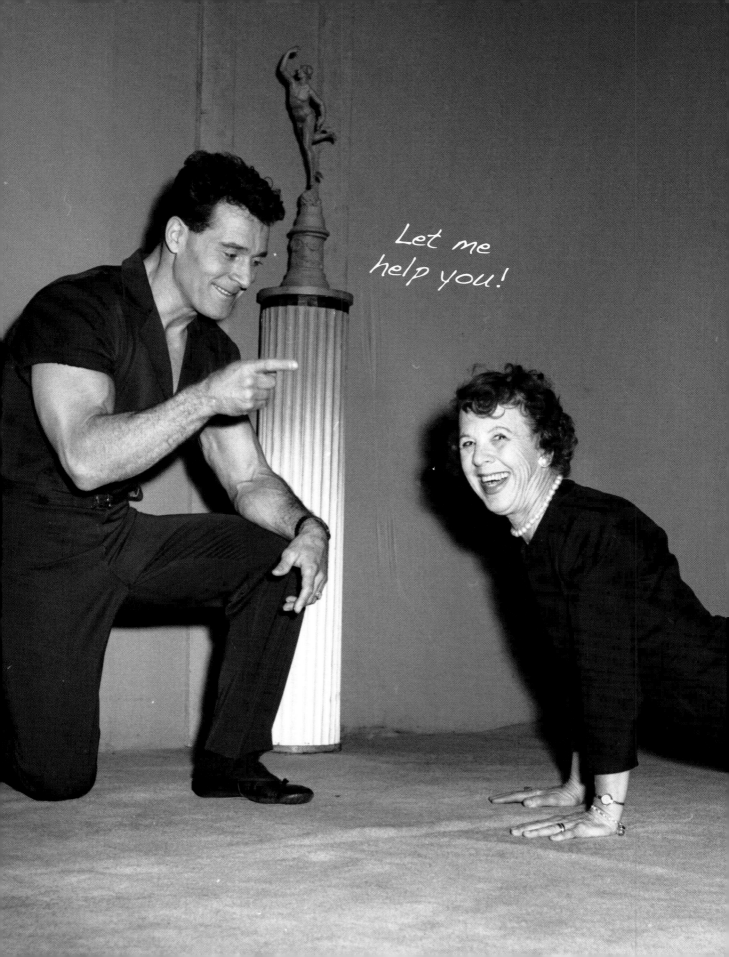

CHAPTER TWO

My Plan For You

LET ME TAKE YOUR HAND

I didn't come from the poorest part of town, but neither were my hardworking parents rolling in money. I have no way of knowing where you come from, what race, how fat or thin, tall or short, what your religion, age, sex or social status happens to be. Nor do I care.

What I care about is your current physical condition and your state of mind.

What I care about is your current physical condition and your state of mind, and my goal is to help you improve both of these to levels beyond your imagination. Way beyond your imagination. The other day an acquaintance asked me if I was an optimist or a pessimist. "Of course I'm an optimist," I said. "I'm planning to live to 120 years of age!" But the truth is that I'm a realist. I've been around people of all weights and sizes, individuals who are fit, energetic and in love with life, and individuals who are sick, depressed and even deathly ill. I'm not a medical doctor. I have a Chiropractic degree and have studied the working of the body my entire life. I can't cure diabetes, cirrhosis, cancer or heart disease, but then nobody can. What I am able to do is help bring you to the healthiest bodyweight and physical condition possible.

I can give you the optimum chance of heading off serious disease by helping you to achieve superior nutrition and to follow a sensible exercise program. There are no guarantees in this life, but we can live our days with healthy activities to get as near to perfect health, fitness and physique as possible. The opposite is to smoke, drink, eat junk food, lie around on the couch and get fat. If any part of this latter account applies to you, then you are not only cutting down on your enjoyment of superior health and vigor, but you have put yourself on a path to an early grave.

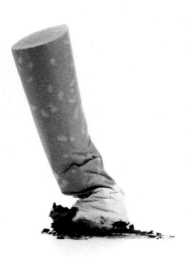

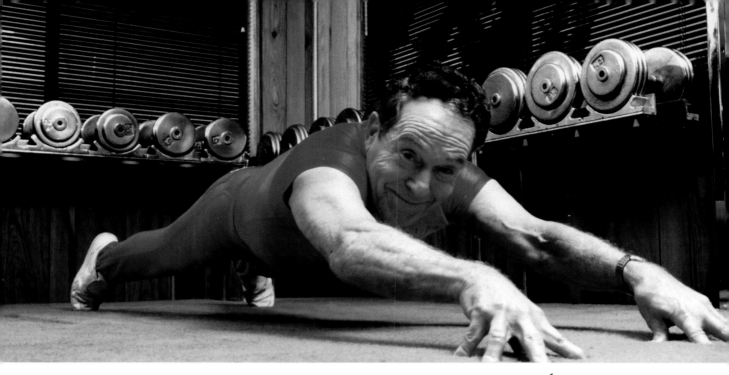

The fact that you have got this far into the text of this book tells me you are serious about making a change in your lifestyle. Well, the rest of your life could indeed be the best years. How do you envision the remainder of your days? Maybe you haven't given it much thought. Will you just keep working, supporting your marriage and children by contributing to the family finances? Have your halfhearted attempts at formal exercise and healthy nutrition caused you to lose that same 20 pounds over and over again? Let me help you reassess your attitude on living. Jump into the happiest, healthiest and most productive years you will ever have.

Remember, I know well of what I speak. I've been a sugarholic. I've been sick from eating junk food. I loved doughnuts, ice cream, and colas. I used to wake up with a headache every morning. I've had bouts of uncontrollable temper, and suffered through illnesses that had me shivering with fear of dying. All this before I was out of my teens. I have no hesitation in letting you know that I believe right now I can make a new person out of you. Whatever your

At age 85, still doing my fingertip pushups.

Jump into the happiest, healthiest and most productive years you will ever have.

age, I can help you change your life. It may seem impossible or at best unlikely, but believe me; you can change your life.

I'll start with your nutritional intake. You may feel there's nothing wrong with the foods we typically eat today: hot dogs and burgers, ice cream, candies, cakes, French fries, doughnuts, gravy, bacon, and fried foods. Your logic says: 'These foods can't be bad, because the government wouldn't allow them to be sold if they were bad.' You've gotta be kidding! The government doesn't care what you eat. Does the president shop for you and pick out your foods? Your local mayor or governor isn't going to do it either. YOU do it! YOU take the initiative and YOU reap the benefits. I know a lot of people say: "If I had the money then I'd be able to achieve health, fitness, peace of mind and joy." I can't say it enough times: your health account and your bank account are synonymous. The more you put in, the more you can take out. You can't buy health and you can't buy fitness. In fact, many millionaires and even billionaires are among the unhappiest and most unhealthy.

You can't buy health and you can't buy fitness.

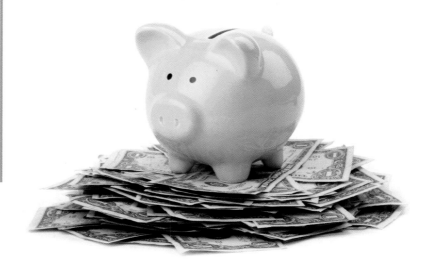

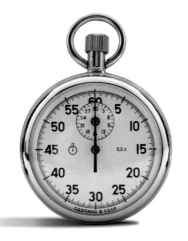

After I get you buying the nutritious foods and passing up on the bad, calorie-dense, sugar-loaded, preservative- and chemically charged foodless merchandise, I'm going to introduce you to formal exercise. Personally, I've been exercising for over 80 years. I'm going to give you the best exercises you can do, either at a gym or in the privacy of your own home. The exercise routine I give you will enable you to tailor it to your own individual strength and fitness levels. There's no all-out strain. No prolonged boring workouts. When you work with the exercises I give you, there is no need to kill yourself straining as though your next gasp of air will be your last. Likewise with the length of your workouts. (Two, three, four hours long enough?) Yeah, right! Your workouts will not exceed 30 or 40 minutes. And you won't even do them every day of the week. I will give you "rest" days, when you don't work out at all. Above all this new plan for your fitness will give you a leg up on longevity. Your joy of living, health and appearance will soar to amazing new levels. Even sex will reach new heights of enjoyment. Did you think I would omit that topic? My plan is to make you marvelously alive.

Yes, I have a plan for you. I'm very serious about getting you to follow it. Why? Because I know that once you have adopted my way of living you will be happier than you've ever been in your life.

As I write these words I'm 95 years of age. No, I'm not as strong or nimble as I was in my younger days; but I'll tell you with all honesty, I don't feel any different than I did as a 25-year-old. I have to repeat that because I want it to sink into your head. *At 95 I don't feel any different than I did at 25.*

How about you?

Don't just gloss over these pages. The information I'm giving you is pure gold. It took me a lifetime to get it all down. Now in a single book you can learn it all. Back in the middle decades of the last century I had a TV exercise program. I was on TV with this show for 35 years. All of North America would tune in and follow me through a workout. I was watched by millions. But I too was a watcher, a watcher of people. All my life I observed others with a keen eye of burning curiosity. I took note of how bums on the street became bums. I noticed the transition of beautiful svelte young bodies as they became ungainly, overweight and deathly sick. I noticed the problems caused by tobacco, alcohol and recreational drugs. I saw literally thousands who went from healthy youth to unhealthy middle age, at which time their unhappy lives were filled with pain and invariably cut short. On the other side of the coin I saw courageous men and women who had given up hope of ever re-shaping their bodies but upon putting forth some effort, gained amazing new health and vitality.

I urge you now. Give me a chance to show you how you really can change your life. Your health, body and expectation of longevity can all be supercharged. Even if you are currently obese and can hardly make it up a flight of stairs, do me this one favor. Let my 95-year-old hand take yours and let you in on what I've learned.

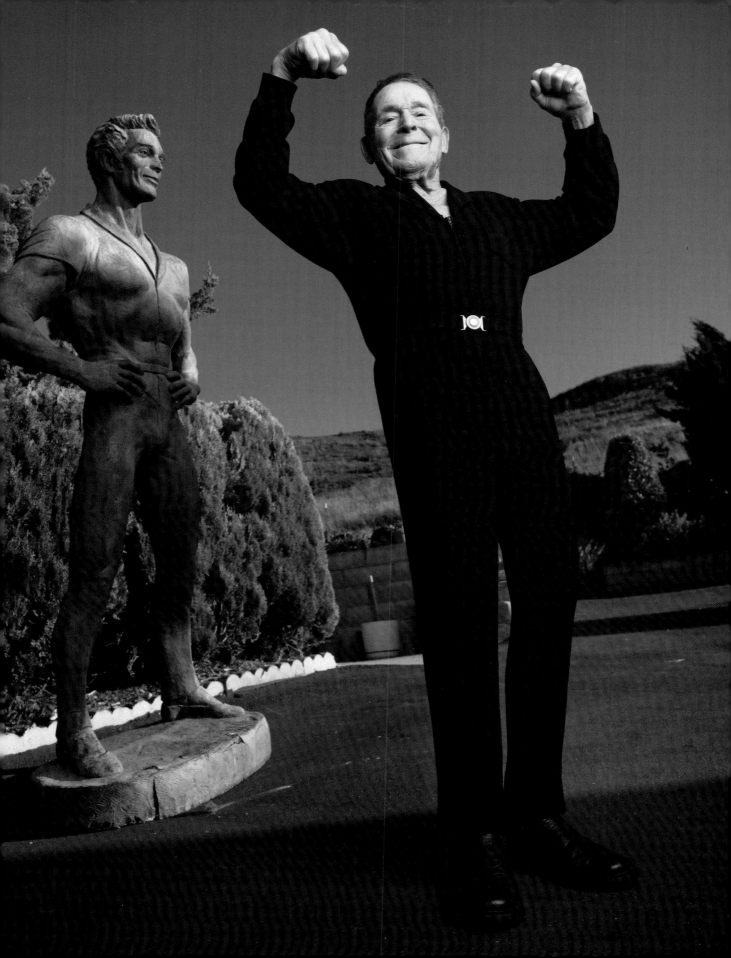

EVERYTHING STARTS WITH A THOUGHT

Isn't it amazing how far man has come in this world? We can see and speak with friends and relations in Australia via our cell phones and computers, and we don't even need any connecting wires. This was impossible just a couple of decades ago. In the past, literally thousands of miles of cable were laid on the seabed, miles below the surface, all to enable us to get a crackly, barely audible voice message across the oceans. Today all we have to do is press a few buttons on our laptops or on our hand-held Black-Berrys, and we're having a face-to-face conversation.

I see scientific and medical progress taking place all around me. But sometimes I wonder how we are doing as human beings. When I take a long hard look around me, I'm not impressed. A recent fact was brought to my attention. It was that children today are not expected to live for as long as their parents. Kinda sad, isn't it? Statistically this means that kids, because of their inactive lifestyles and poor eating habits, will not live to the age their parents will likely live. Of course there will be exceptions, but the point is clear. Good health and good intellect are the two greatest blessings in life. If you are born with health, as most of us are, you have hope. And if you have hope you have everything.

If you have hope you have everything.

The health of the people within a nation is an almost unfailing index of its morals. The health of those people is also an indication of the potential of the economy of that nation. America would be more prosperous if its health rate were higher. Most of us openly admire those individuals who are fit and strong, so why are we all so depressed as a nation? Why is illness on the rise? Why are we a nation of super obese? The loss to the country through unnecessary illnesses is enormous. I believe that if we follow the steps in this book, our life expectancy could be hugely increased to many more years above current average longevity expectation.

Men and women should live longer. They should also be getting more joy out of every day and the adventures that day brings. "To preserve health," said Samuel Johnson, the English literary genius, "is a moral and religious duty, for health is the basis of all social virtues. We no longer can be useful when not well."

Without health where is the joy in life? Too many people are unaware in matters of health, fitness, exercise and nutrition and it is reaching tremendous proportions. And look how many people try and make money from it. Check out any drug store and look at the scores of products that are supposed to help us eliminate better, beat stomachaches, relieve heartburn, stop diarrhea, cure headaches, lose weight, overcome skin problems, varicose veins, bad breath, hypertension and fatigue. You name it.

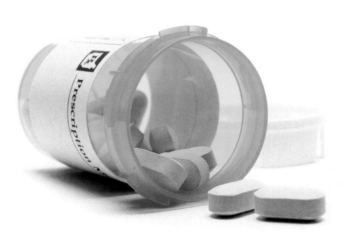

People spend billions on pills and drugs that have no real benefit.

I had lots of problems as a 14-year-old. I had headaches, skin eruptions, nervousness, bad breath and who knows what else. But I wised up and made changes. I discovered exercise and good nutrition, and have enjoyed a pain-free, energy-filled life ever since.

Americans spend billions upon billions of dollars on tobacco, booze and junk food, and then spend billions more on drugs that have no real benefit. The American Medical Association estimates that the sale of reducing remedies, pain and headache relievers, sleeping pills and tranquilizers cost Americans a substantial part of their wages every week.

There is no doubt that millions of men and women are living far below their best level of physical fitness. We are all in agreement that our health is important, yet health is not valued until sickness comes. Doctors agree with me that most of the causes of dying before one's time are avoidable. We are simply ignorant and careless about our wellness factor.

I have written this book because I want you to experience the same joy of living that I have. I'm not exaggerating when I say that when I built up my health with proper exercise and superior nutrition, every day was a joy. I mean it. Every day. And it's still that way. Sure I'm going to die one day. That happens to all of us. But isn't it exciting to know we can push the barriers and regain the health, strength and energy of our younger years? Follow the stages in this book and I will lead you to happier and longer days. After all, I did do it for myself, right?

I want you to experience the same joy of living that I have.

Don't make the mistake of thinking money is everything. Health and fitness are way more important. There is no wealth like health, because wealth can't buy health. But when you have

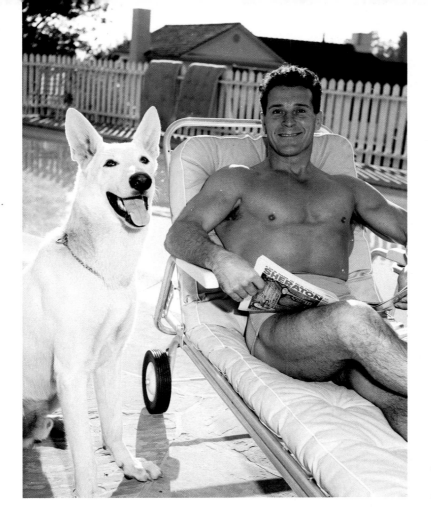

There is no wealth like health!

health you have vitality, and so your ambition and passion for making money can be set free. Wealth without health is a mockery. The healthy laborer is better off than a sick millionaire. But believe me, if you are a fit and energy-filled person who is bubbling with wellness, you can apply yourself to any career that takes your fancy. And that career, together with the money it commands, will come to you faster because your enthusiasm for the job will be fired up by your superior physical fitness.

Okay, so I have planted the thought in your mind. You want to be fitter and healthier. You want to feel great all day. You want to live an energy-filled lifestyle, and you want to live to a ripe old age. Let's go.

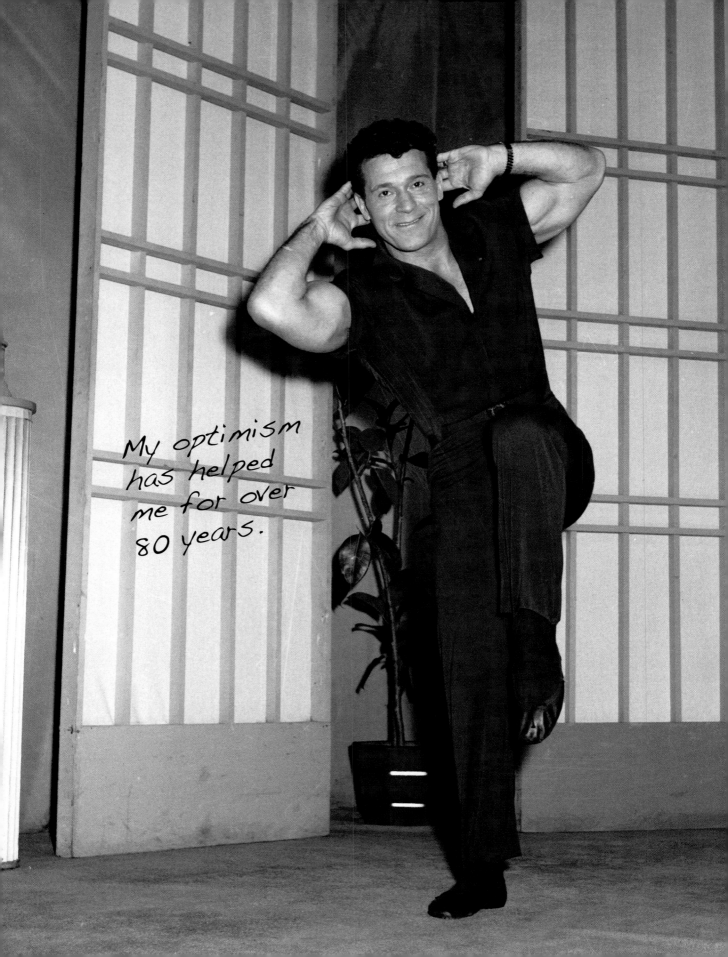

My optimism
has helped
me for over
80 years.

CHAPTER THREE

Far From Perfect

WE'RE ONLY HUMAN

> I can't wait to get out of bed in the morning and greet the new day.

The rest of your life is the best of your life! So get a calendar and circle the date. The rest of your life awaits … and this is the first day. Anybody who knows me knows I bubble over with enthusiasm. I can't wait to get out of bed in the morning and greet the new day. But it wasn't always that way. Even though I have worked on my body, mind and personality for some 80 years, I am far from perfect. I have had my own mishaps and disappointments. In my last year at Berkeley High School in California, I underwent a serious operation on my right knee as a result of a football injury. I was on crutches for months, unable to walk without assistance. My doctor was very negative in his prognosis, and when I questioned him repeatedly he finally admitted that walking on my own was not a future likelihood.

I was shocked at my doctor's prognosis. I had never considered for one minute that I wouldn't walk again. After giving the situation serious thought I decided that even though I couldn't put one foot in front of the other I would master the art of walking by progressive degrees of effort. I finally managed a few steps and then with enormous optimism (which must have come from my naturally stubborn nature) I found the steepest hill in Berkeley, my hometown, and made up my mind that one day I would make it to the top. Each day I would walk a little further than I had the day before and after several months I finally made it to the top. This was in 1933 and I was 19.

Even though I could now walk and climb hills I was unable to do a full squat. But I worked hard at every other form of exercise, including wrestling, swimming, hand balancing and martial arts. I

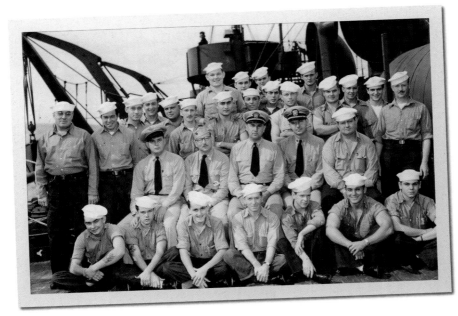

My Naval crewman and me. I'm 2nd from the right in the bottom row.

loved bodybuilding and wanted to build a Mr. America-type physique. When World War II broke out I tried to enlist, but was 4F because I was unable to do a full squat. I tried repeatedly in various branches of the military. After several failures I went with a high-school buddy, Al Markstein, who was born on the very same day as me, and was enlisting in the navy. As I was going through the line I did handstands, one-arm pushups and many of my balancing tricks. I so captivated the examining doctor that he forgot to ask me to do the compulsory squat and gave me an A1 grade. I found out later that this examining doctor was the surgeon who had operated on my knee seven years earlier.

Much later, when I was 68, an out-of-control truck hit my car head-on. My good left knee went into the dashboard and I had to have another operation. So you see, we all have physical problems of one kind or another. Truth is, I've yet to see a perfect human being. But that shouldn't stop us from aiming to be as fit, strong and healthy as possible.

We all have physical problems of one kind or another.

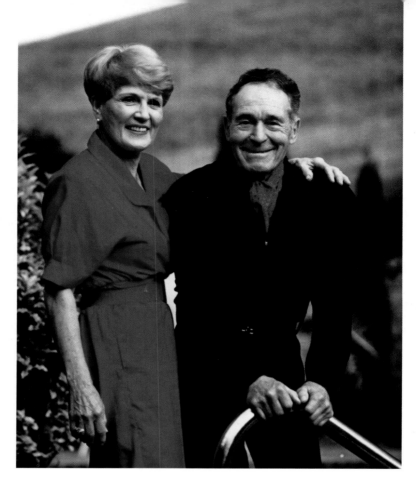

My wife Elaine and I
at home in California.

Elaine, my wife, also suffered as a result of an accident. She was stopped at a traffic light when a bus with failing brakes ran into the back of her. The impact ruptured the gas tank and sent her skidding into traffic from the Hollywood Bowl. Her whole right side was severely wrenched and she suffered an extreme whiplash. In spite of persistent pain she continued with exercise and therapy, which included a solid nutrition program. Today at well over 80 she says she's pain free and going on 29.

Where are you today? Are you 40, 50 or 60 or older? Have you climbed into your dotage already? What is old age, anyway? I'll tell you. Old age is someone 20 years older than you are. For me that is someone around 115. For a 60-year-old it is 80. For an 80-year-old it's 100. Not a bad philosophy is it?

Old age is someone 20 years older than you are.

The other day someone asked me what age I wanted to live to. I answered: *I can't die; it would ruin my image!* That brought a laugh. The truth is, of course, if I died tomorrow I would have no regrets. My life has been full and rewarding. I have enjoyed every second of my life since discovering the fitness lifestyle. Most important to me is the fact that I have been able to help so many see the light. Fitness guru Richard Simmons paid me a compliment: "Thanks, Jack. It may have taken a while but it looks like the country finally got the message – including me! There's not a single person in the world of fitness who doesn't owe you a salute."

And Robert Kennedy, the publisher of *MuscleMag International, Oxygen, Reps!,* and *Maximum Fitness,* says quite simply that he started his publishing empire because he was influenced by seeing me on my TV series the first day he landed on North American shores from the UK way back in 1966.

> **I can't die; it would ruin my image!**

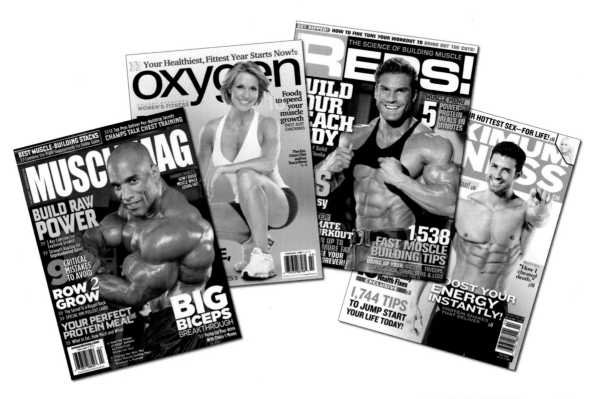

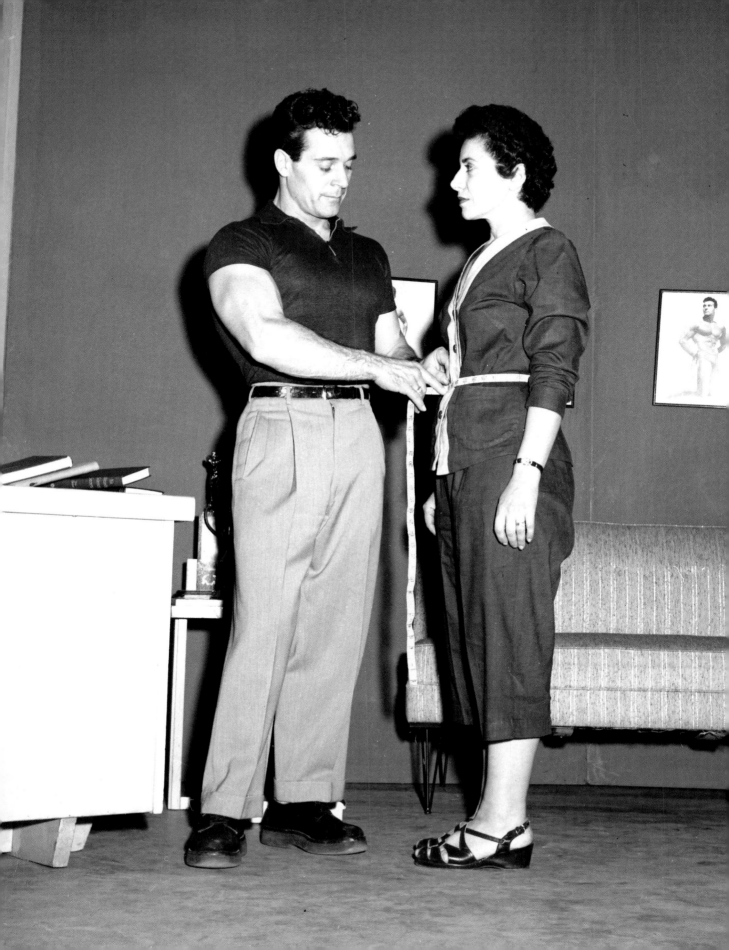

When I look back on my career and close my eyes I can see and hear so many comments by friends and acquaintances. Some good; some bad. I have helped so many who are eternally grateful but here have been some who have fallen through the cracks. Regrettably, my loving father was one of them. I was still a senior in high school and my friend Freddy Nelson and I were headed for a weekend at the Russian River. We were excited at the thought of romping on the beach, swimming and dancing the night away in the evenings.

When I was ready to leave that morning Dad was waiting at the bottom of the stairs. "I don't feel too good," he said. "Can you drop me off at the doctor's on your way to Russian River?" At that time Dad was in his early 40s, no longer the svelte dancing coach who had met my mother on the ship from France. He had fallen, as had most men of his age, into typical middle-aged habits, careless about his food and showing no interest in formal exercise. At five feet five, he weighed 185 pounds. Far too much for a man of his height. Because of his habit of eating only foods that tasted good to him in combination with his negligence over exercise, his waist was paunchy and his chest had slipped. His arms were scrawny and his entire muscular structure had atrophied into a sea of flab. At an age when he could have been a dynamic, virile man, he had let it all go by neglect.

I loved my Dad like crazy, but his main trouble was that he ate the wrong foods, and he ate too much. I tried to get him to exercise and eat sensibly but he didn't see anything wrong with his lifestyle, and after all I was "just a kid," what did I know?

Like most men Dad ate some good foods, but he spoiled

> **He ate the wrong foods, and he ate too much.**

> **My own father was helplessly struggling to suck air inside an oxygen tank.**

them. For example, he liked salads but ruined them with gobs of fatty, calorie-dense dressings. He loved French bread spread thick with butter and thick slices of cheese, and he had to take numerous cups of coffee throughout the day, loaded with cream and sugar. His evenings were spent sitting in his chair listening to the radio till all hours, and before going to bed he'd have more junk food, or what he called "a little snack." Perhaps you have someone like my Dad in your family? (You know all the trips to the kitchen for a seltzer, soda or beer.) The shortness of breath climbing stairs. It's all too common.

That summer day we crossed to San Francisco on the ferry. Freddy and I were laughing about our plans for fun once we reached the river. Dad said little. He wasn't a complainer by nature. Perhaps he felt that his physicality was on a downward curve. Many men feel this in the privacy of their minds yet do nothing positive to change things around.

We dropped Dad off and headed up through the redwoods to the river, where life and youth were joined in endless fun and antics. At the end of the weekend I got the call. Dad wasn't expected to live. Hurrying back to San Francisco I couldn't believe my eyes. My own father, helplessly struggling to suck air inside an oxygen tank. He was gaunt and grey, hardly recognizable. He'd had a coronary attack. They also found cirrhosis. As always he didn't complain, but this time he couldn't. He couldn't talk. Only the tear in his eyes, unforgettable, told of his regrets. That night he was gone. The death of my gentle Dad is why I am a health crusader today.

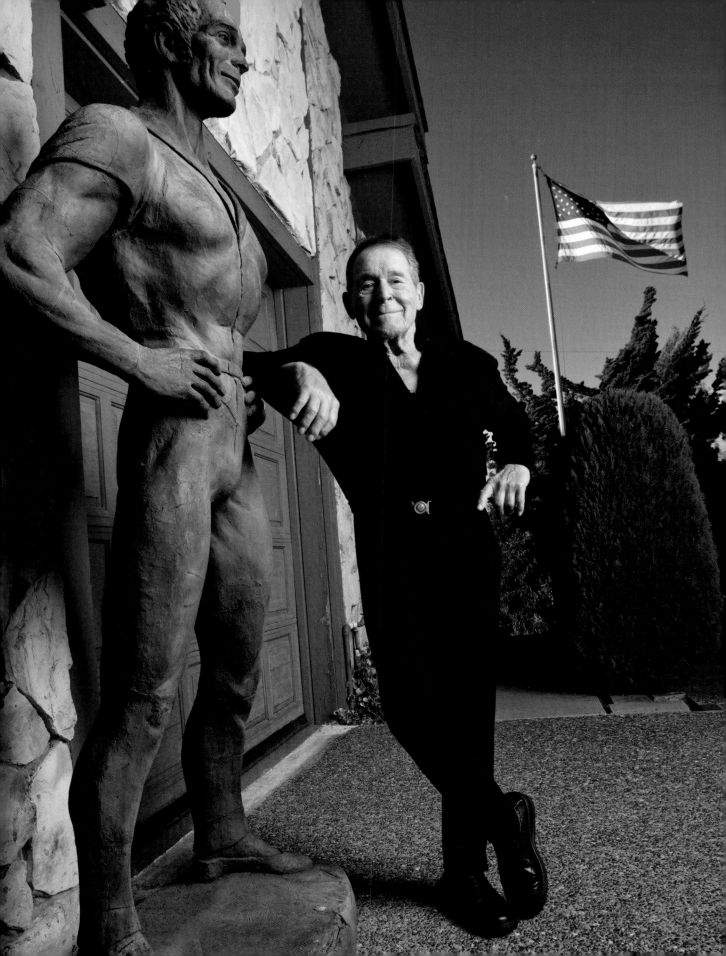

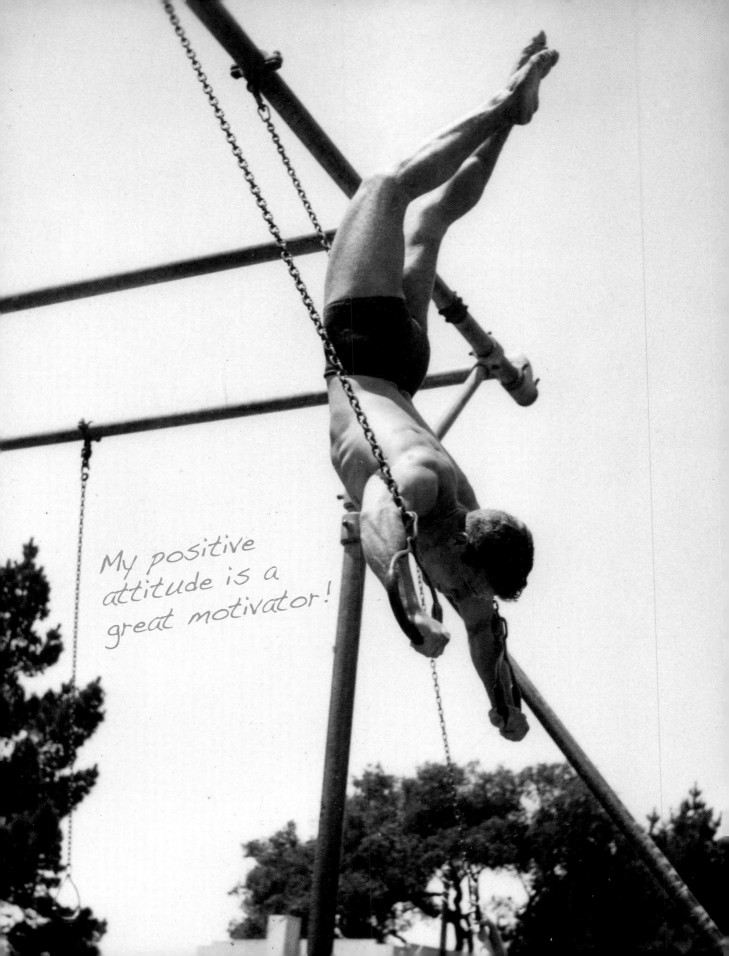

My positive
attitude is a
great motivator!

CHAPTER FOUR

Step 1: Motivation

YOUR ESSENTIAL STARTING POINT

Being motivated is a wonderful gift. It really is. As long as I can remember I was always passionate. I wanted to be a somebody. I didn't know what, and I certainly didn't know how. My self-esteem was in the toilet, but even though I was an undersized skinny teenager I would hyperventilate from the need to be successful, famous or of use to the world. I was ready, willing and able, but my life was a daily struggle and nothing on the horizon held any promise. Not, that is, until I found the solution was in following a systematic program of exercise and proper nutrition.

Today I get scores of e-mails from individuals who claim to have no motivation. "I need you to kick my butt" is a very common phrase they use. When I ask exactly what their problem is, most of the answers I get follow a similar pattern: "I used to be slim, but then I let myself go." "I try to lose weight but never stick to the diet." "If I join a gym I seldom go more than half a dozen times before quitting." "I have lost the same 10 pounds over and over again, but I really need to lose 50. I can't stay motivated." Do any of these sound familiar to you?

A lack of motivation is a hard nut to crack. We can approach the subject in numerous ways. One could use the fear tactic: If you don't quit tobacco, eat healthier and exercise you'll get fat and have a stroke. And then there's the lost romance warning: How can you expect to find a decent partner in life if you don't even take care of yourself? And what about this one: When you have a great body you not only have better health and fitness, but you feel special. People stop you in grocery stores to ask your secret.

When you have a great body you not only have better health and fitness, but you feel special.

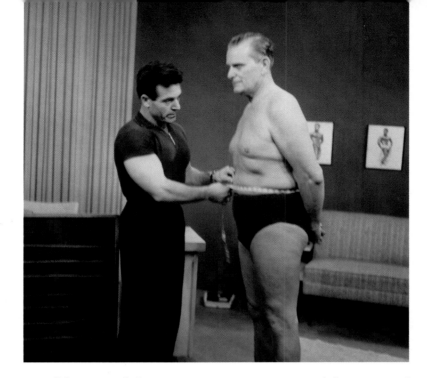

Helping people lose weight on The Jack LaLanne Show.

Of course all these scenarios carry some truth but my usual suggestion is that the person lacking motivation take some quiet time to themselves and find a full-length mirror. Lock the door and disrobe. That's right. Strip off all your clothes. Don't smile and flex your shoulders. No sucking in that gut! Relax that tummy. Now stand sideways. Come on, let it all hang out. Now, this is the real you. Happy?

Continue to relax. Continue to be self-critical. Get mad at yourself. How could you let this happen to your body? You were born with the greatest gift of all: physical health. So why are you continuing to let it get away? This is the time to answer the question: Are you going to continue as you have, clogging your arteries, and adding layers of fat to every part of your body, risking ill health, aches and pains and an early grave? Or are you going to devote the rest of your life to being fit, feeling eternally great and eating only healthy nutrition that will not only keep you tight and lean but will stand you in good stead to live for longer than the average person?

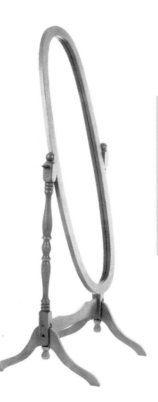

Check yourself out
in the mirror; relax
the body, and get mad.

In my case I didn't have a second's pause. I knew what I wanted and I never regretted one minute of working out or following a clean diet. I should add here that my suggestion of stripping off in front of a full-length mirror and getting mad at one's image has been criticized. The argument being that I am lowering people's self esteem even more. I do sympathize with this point of view, but tough love is sometimes the only way to get people to commit. Forgive me if I have offended you.

Over the years I have motivated literally millions of men and women, and hopefully men and women not yet born will benefit from my teachings. But not all of those I inspired followed through with a lifetime commitment. When revisiting some of these individuals I found through almost 80 years of trial and error that I had to get serious with some people. I needed to spell out that their drinking problem was damaging their organs; that their daily pack of cigarettes would one day turn their lungs black with cancer; that their obesity and high cholesterol would close off their arteries one by one … until a crippling stroke would put them in a wheelchair or a coffin. When gentle persuasion fails, tough love may be the only answer.

How do we keep motivated? Reading magazines and books on the subject can be motivating. Personally I enjoy Robert Kennedy's *Oxygen* magazine, devoted to women's fitness. And for men, his *Maximum Fitness* magazine deals with training and nutrition. Study the photographs of fit men and women. You too can look that amazing. Just checking out an image can make you want to run to the gym.

Me with some of the crew at KGO-TV.

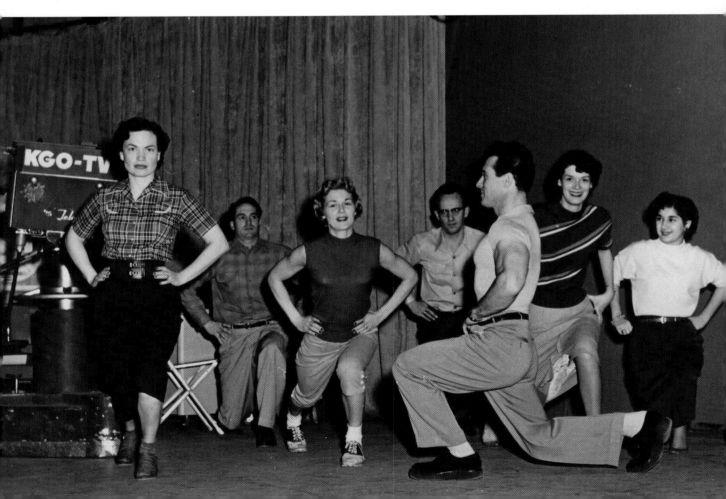

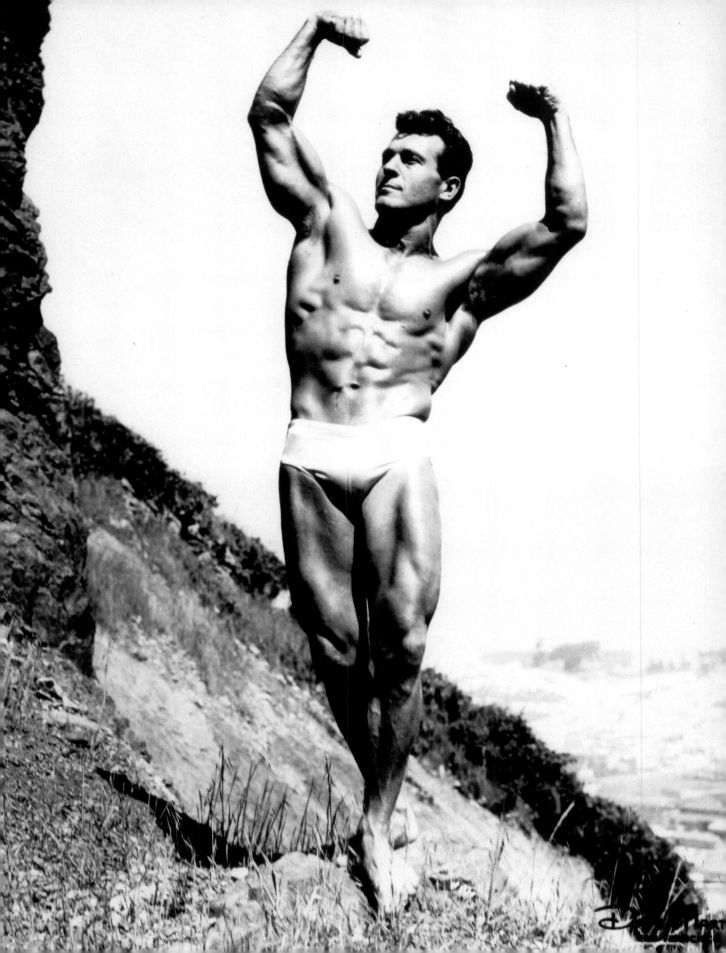

Not in a relationship right now? What better motivation to get into the best shape of your life! Ditto for weddings, high school and family reunions. Just remember to keep up with your new lifestyle after these events are history.

What is the greatest motivator of all? Let me tell you a story. When I started weight training, I of course wanted instant results. The only thing that happened was that my muscles were sore. After squatting I could hardly walk; after bench pressing my chest and arms ached for days ... I had my doubts about the efficacy of lifting weights. Then after three weeks I looked in my bathroom mirror and I saw bigger pectorals, triceps and even an improved V-taper in my back. My passion for, and belief in, weight training soared! Seeing your own progress is the greatest motivator of all.

For some reason I love motivating people. I still do it on tele-vision, selling my juicer. Why? Because I believe in juicing and I have confidence that my juicer is a fantastic buy. I used this same enthusiasm when encouraging people to join my health club. And then when I had my own salespeople I would tell them: "All I'm asking you to do is sign up a man or a woman to a year or two year membership; explain that they get much more out of it than the money we get out of it. I'm not asking you to twist arms, or sell a fake muscle-building tonic. Just go out there and help people look and feel better. They'll love you for it!" Believe me that little speech helped.

Seeing your own progress is the greatest motivator of all.

HOW TO
STAY MOTIVATED

→ Check yourself out in the mirror, relax the body and get mad.

→ Read books and magazines that have inspiring photos and great articles.

→ Tell yourself to eat well and exercise for well-being and longevity.

→ Break bad habits. No tobacco, alcohol or drugs to interfere with your commitment.

→ Get a training partner so you can keep each other stimulated and on track.

→ Organize your day so that you have time to exercise and eat correctly.

→ Develop a positive attitude. Think and picture how amazing you are going to be. Visualize it!

→ Take a photo of yourself and stick it on the fridge or bathroom mirror.

→ Set an achievable goal for yourself and be totally committed to following through.

→ Build a "worse case scenario" picture in your mind. Do you really want things to deteriorate to this degree?

→ Whether your prime interest is in being fit, living longer or having a sexually appealing figure, keep your target front and center.

→ Recognize that willpower has to be nurtured. You can mentally rev up your engine of commitment.

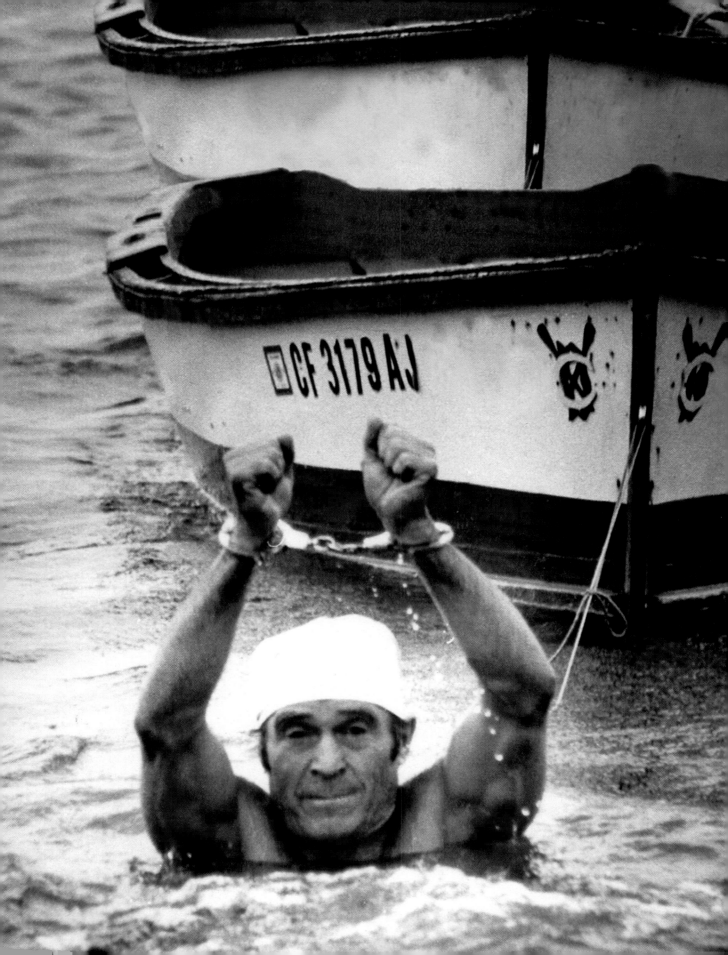

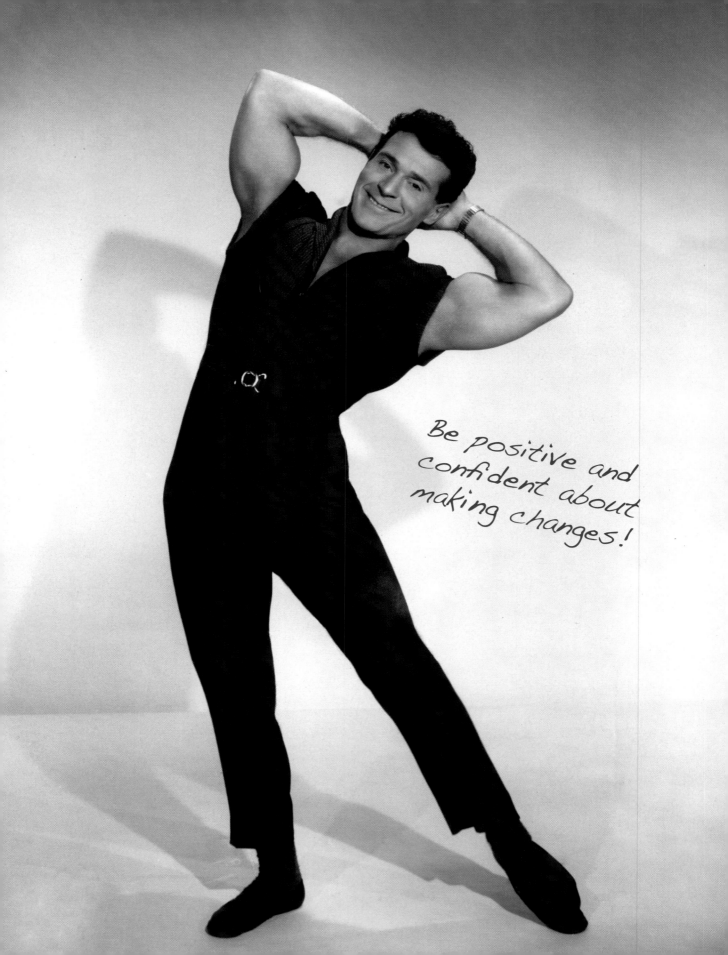

Be positive and confident about making changes!

CHAPTER FIVE

Step 2: Step Away From Killer Habits

COMMIT YOURSELF

Okay, so we are ready to get started. Come with me to that full-length mirror in your bedroom. Let's take a long hard look. Stand sideways. Relax the tummy. Are we impressed by our current condition, mildly disappointed, or downright shocked to the core at how we have let ourselves go?

And how old are you? Thirty, 40, 50 … or getting up there to 60, 70, 80? Whatever your age – and admittedly this is a bit of a hassle – you are going to have to get a physical checkup. So get on the phone and make an appointment with your professional healthcare provider. It's always best before changing your nutritional or exercise habits to get your doctor's okay. Ask for a stress test. It's no big deal. When your doctor hears that you intend on starting an exercise program and eating healthier foods, chances are he will be delighted. After the checkup is complete and you have the green light to go ahead with your new lifestyle, you too will be delighted. By all means show this book to your doctor.

I have no way of telling if you are fat or thin, tall or short, young or not so young. Neither do I know to what degree, if any, you have let yourself go. Looking around I am saddened by the indolence and indifference of the average North American and the ease with which he has permitted himself to slide. This has now become a world-wide phenomenon. There has been a shocking overindulgence in the so-called good life, along with inactivity, the unsound habit of poor nutrition, and the body- and mind-destroying habits involving tobacco, recreational drugs and alcohol. Our first step then is to clean house of our health-

Whatever your age you are going to have to get a physical checkup.

destroying habits. Be positive and confident about making these changes. So many people expect failure; and when they do, they are seldom disappointed.

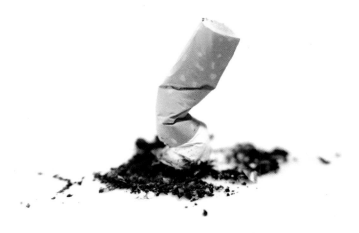

SMOKING

If you are a cigarette, pipe or cigar smoker, stop now. I can think of nothing more damaging you could do to the soft tissue of the body. Not just the lungs and throat are weakened and ultimately pulverized by the heat and chemicals of smoke, but tobacco smoking poisons the blood, cells and organs of the body. There is not any part of your physical body, skin, eyes, hair, or even your nails that are not severely damaged by smoking. Smoking kills because the poisons from smoke get into the bloodstream, and the blood goes everywhere.

We usually experiment with smoking in our teens. It's the "grown-up" thing to do. One's first cigarette is inevitibly a cough-inducing horror story, invariably followed by a session of vomiting. Does that tell you something? The second attempt usually comes when friends light up and offer you a cigarette. Your mind says,

You are aware that smoking is bad for you. Quit this minute!

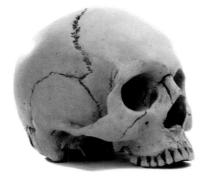

> **Smoking will contribute to an early demise.**

"Why not? I've done this before. I'll show my friends I can smoke with the best of 'em." Before you know it, you're a regular smoker. And not long after you're well and truly hooked.

Now you have a problem. You are aware that smoking is bad for you. You thought you couldn't get addicted. Now you've tried to quit a few times, but weakened and gave up the battle. You're almost resigned to smoking for the rest of your life. It's not that you really enjoy it. You just find that you *need* it! My advice right now — and I mean this with every fiber of my body — is to quit this minute. Take your cigarettes out of the pack, screw them up in your hands and flush them down the toilet. Never for one second allow yourself even one puff of a cigarette again in your lifetime. During the next few weeks you will be tempted. Oh, how you'll be tempted! The first few days will be hell. But do not give in. Do you hear me? Do *not* give in! I promise you after a few weeks you will no longer feel the urge to smoke. In fact when anyone smokes within 20 yards you will wave your hands in front of your face and extol with annoyance, "Who's smoking? Please, not near me. It chokes me up!"

One last time — smoking is lethal. It will make you short of breath. It will rob you of energy. It will make you sick. It will shorten your life by contributing to an early, painful demise. Stop today!

DRUGS

There are so many drugs today, one hardly knows where to begin. The big drug companies are constantly trying to get you onto some kind of drug therapy, for the rest of your life. Just imagine the millions upon millions of North Americans who have been persuaded to be on a never-ending drug program. And then what happens? You turn the television on and there's this lawyer's group running an ad, "If you've taken so-and-so prescription drug and have suffered side effects please contact us. We may be able to get you a settlement." And then they go on to say, "Contact us even if you haven't suffered any side effects." All this raises the question: If the drugs are harming us, why were they given the green light in the first place?

Don't get me wrong. There are useful drugs out there. Drugs that relieve pain. Drugs that can save your life. But in general the medical world has gone prescription-drug crazy. Many people are permanently on a half dozen drugs all the time. Ideally, we shouldn't need any drugs. Our cholesterol levels, heart rhythms,

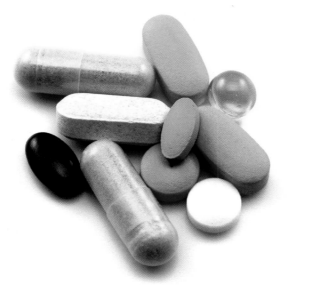

The big drug companies are constantly trying to get you onto some kind of drug therapy.

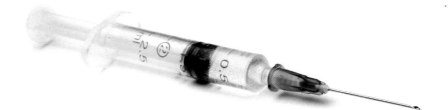

energy output, blood pressure, organ function, body-fat levels and whatever else you could mention should all be in healthy working order. But because of our lazy lives and terrible eating habits we put ourselves into a state of unhealthiness. Today we know a thousand times more about diseases than our predecessors did generations ago, but apparently we know infinitely less about health. The greatest challenge of public health today is keeping the middle-aged physically fit.

Then there are the so-called "recreational" drugs. When I hear the statistics of the hundreds of thousands of Americans of all ages who are on recreational drugs, from ecstasy and cocaine to crystal-meth and heroin … I just shake my head. It's not just rampant in the showbiz world of acting and music, but is in every corner of the American continent, from the big cities to the smallest country towns. Drugs often start at house parties, nightclubs or social get togethers. If you've never been involved with recreational drugs, say no when the day comes you are offered. I have seen good friends become social misfits through drugs, unable to work or interact normally with other humans. Drugs are known to make people forget their problems; to feel better, to enjoy a "high," but all highs are followed by lows. At their conclusion these lows become nightmares that will take you to the absolute depths of personal pain and suffering. And ultimately to a predisposition to crime, ill health, an unbalanced mind and untimely death. Stay clear, my friend.

Drugs become nightmares that will take you to the absolute depths of pain and suffering.

COFFEE AND ALCOHOL ABUSE

I was once called a health nut. When I opened my first gymnasium word got around that this loony Frenchman, Jack LaLanne, was charging people to exercise. Today there are still health nuts around who are totally against the consumption of both coffee and alcohol. They regard it as a cardinal sin. I am not one of those people. I don't hold with those who say coffee is terrible, though I don't drink it myself. As for alcohol, I will have a glass of wine or champagne on occasions. I never lose control of my drinking, frequently only having half, rather than a full glass. I do of course recognize that both excessive coffee and especially alcohol consumption can be dangerous temptations for some people. Alcohol is concentrated sugar. But it is an addictive sugar and many hundreds of thousands of Americans have become alcoholics, unable to work or even function in any way approaching normality. They become slaves to drink and frequently find themselves destitute, and on the streets living in soup kitchens, and spending any money begged from the public on more alcohol, and the inevitable cigarettes. Even if they don't get to this point, their lives and families will often be destroyed. Drinking has to be controlled. Small amounts have not been shown to be harmful. Large amounts have been known to kill.

Many Americans have become alcoholics with lives and families often destroyed.

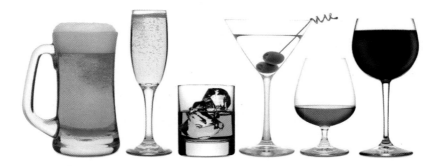

Coffee is not in the same category. But like alcohol, excessive consumption can make us sick. Because of the preponderance of coffee houses, drive thrus, break trucks that visit businesses throughout the day, and coffee machines, this popular stimulant is accessible 24/7. Many office workers have a coffee on the go at their desks throughout their entire 9-to-5 work hours. But first they have a couple of cups at breakfast. Then they buy a coffee on their way to work and again when they leave. Too much coffee can upset our stomachs, and because it is a stimulant its consumption can lead to anxiety, stress and overall nervousness. Again, it is the excess that harms us.

Too much coffee can upset our stomachs and lead to anxiety, stress and overall nervousness.

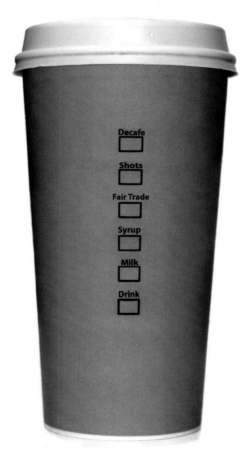

STRESSED OUT

Right off the bat, ginseng is widely acknowledged as helping the body cope with stress. So are vitamins B1 and B3. But what is stress, anyway? Defined, it is the accumulated effect of ongoing concern for things that have happened, are happening, or are suspected to be about to happen. Stress builds up over a variety of emotions, including anger, jealousy, greed, revenge – you name it. People get stressed because of their poor health, overwork, lack of sleep, disorderliness, aging, worry over finances and annoying habits of a spouse. I have learned the things we worry so much

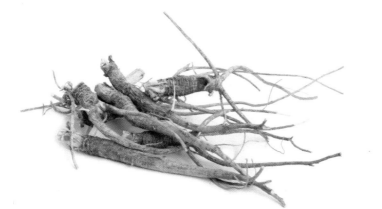

Ginseng is widely acknowledged as helping the body cope with stress.

about seldom materialize, especially if we take action to solve the matters at hand.

As a pre-teen and early teenager, I was hugely stressed. I firmly believe it was killing me. I was a skinny fellow with excessively low self-esteem; I had a face full of acne and had constant stomachache from daily worry. I wanted to be a somebody, but felt like a nobody. It was only after I changed my lifestyle to healthy nutrition and regular strenuous exercise that stress left me, never to return.

Make no mistake about it; stress is a killer. It is one of the most common maladies in the U.S.A. Literally millions of North Americans take painkillers or drink alcohol in order to relax their minds artificially so stress will be less destructive of their bodies. This leads to addiction and of course stress is further worsened when the addiction is finally mastered.

How do we beat stress? The answer lies in the basic premise of this book. Exercise and diet. Regular strenuous workouts will pluck away those pangs of stress, and a seven-day-a-week diet of whole foods, nutrition in its natural state, not remanufactured by the inept hand of man, will go a long way to helping relieve stress.

I believe the reason I don't have a high degree of stress is because I have kept myself busy all my life. I have tackled situations head-on rather than put myself into a state of stress with constant worry when problems arrive. Curiously, when it comes to public speaking, which I still do on a regular basis, I seek a certain degree of stress. But I prepare my speeches with great care. I always make sure I know six times more about my subject than my audience does, but I welcome a degree of nervousness (stress) before I step up on stage. It keeps me sharp. My heart is working a little overtime and my breathing is a tad faster. My brain and mouth are well oiled and my seminars and speaking engagements invariably bring the house down. It's all about passion for doing things right, isn't it?

I welcome a degree of nervousness before I step up on stage. It keeps me sharp.

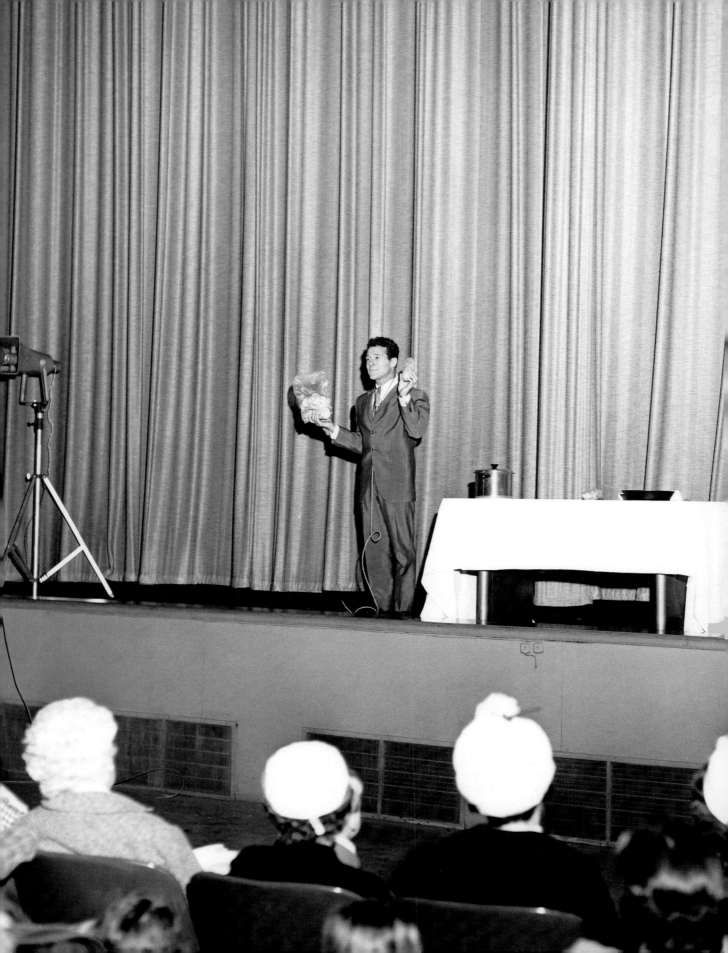

GUIDE TO
REDUCING STRESS

→ Be prepared for the unexpected.

→ Don't take a job of which you know little, are careless about, or that you find extremely difficult.

→ Don't expect constant approval at work or in the home. It seldom materializes.

→ Work out at least three days a week: weights, stretching, walking, treadmill, yoga, Pilates.

→ Prioritize your "to-do list" and follow through in order of importance.

→ Eat clean: Natural, wholesome foods. Plenty of fruit and vegetables, whole grains, lean protein.

→ Don't worry about the future; plan your future. Set achievable goals, and follow through.

→ Do everything that is healthy for your mind and body. No junk food, drugs, or cigarettes, and very limited alcohol.

→ Delegate some of your workload to others; you cannot do everything.

→ Learn to completely relax at different times of the day. Put your feet up and watch a half-hour TV comedy program or read a good book.

→ Don't chase massive wealth or actively seek happiness through possessions. Happiness comes from within.

→ Find a strong relationship. Develop reliable, solid friends and be loyal.

→ If someone cuts you off on the highway, or if a friend, coworker or family member gives you a scowl or shows aggression, ignore it. Let no one, and I mean no one, ruin your day.

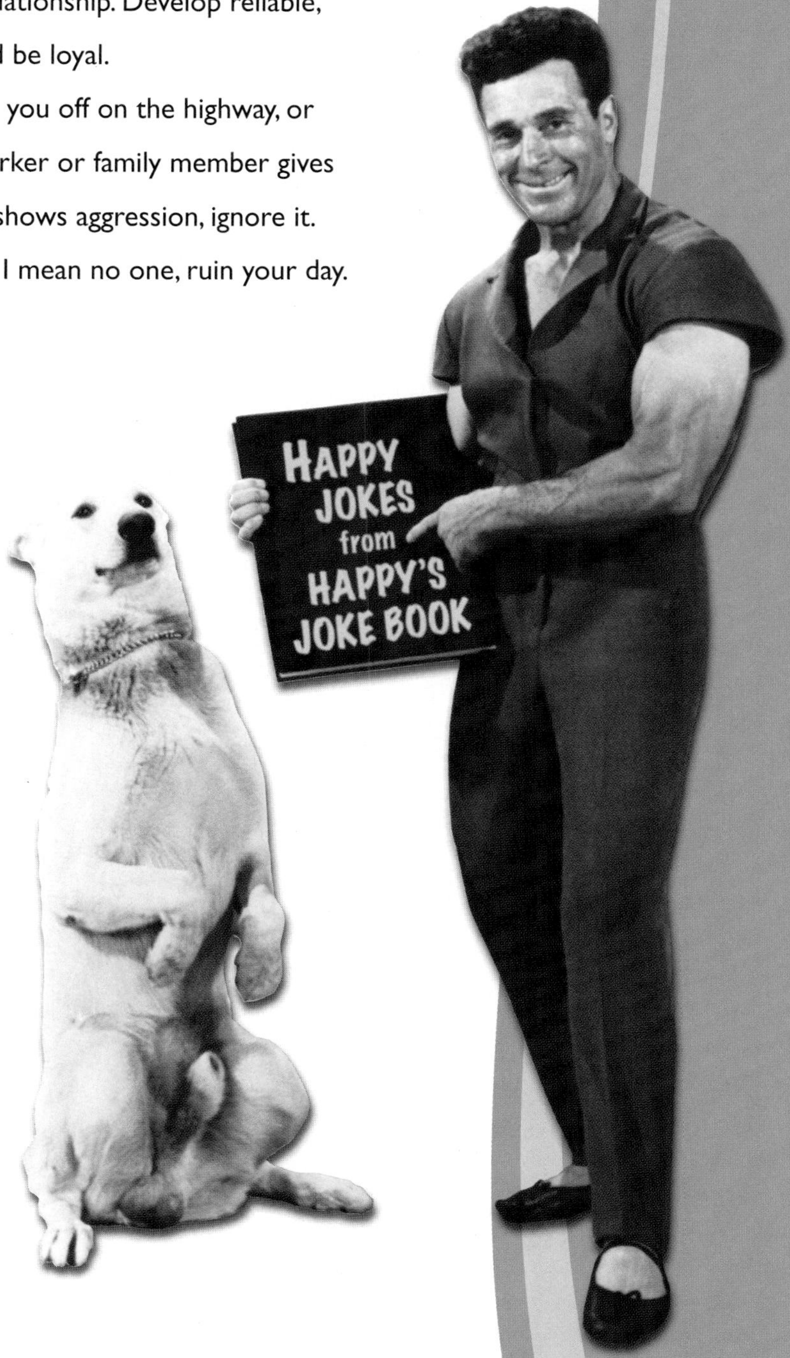

HAPPY
JOKES
from
HAPPY'S
JOKE BOOK

Good habits are the key to success!

CHAPTER SIX

Step 3:
Personal Care

FEELING FRESH, HEALTHY AND ATTRACTIVE

We can't do much about the face we inherited from our ancestors, but we can make the most of what we've got. My "thing" has always been about proper nutrition, vigorous exercise and developing passion for life. But there's more to it than that.

In this day and age one wouldn't think it necessary to talk about personal care, hygiene and general appearance, but truth to tell many people don't take care of themselves as they should. And it's seldom because of lack of money. Admittedly the street bum is not going to easily climb out of his dilemma, shower and change his socks and underwear on a daily basis, but sloppy personal habits are not the exclusive domain of the financially broken. Good hygiene is not just about smelling good and wearing clean clothes. It's very much about happiness. And about the longevity that comes with living a clean, healthy life. Good habits are the key to success. Poor habits unlock the door to failure.

SHOWERING

Taking a daily shower is an important part of my day. What is it they say? Cleanliness is next to Godliness? Scientists believe that body odor is like the appendix, a vestige of our evolution. That is, the smells we give off from our bodies, namely the armpits and the groin, may have once served to proclaim our sexuality.

Good hygiene is not just about smelling good and being clean, but it's very much about happiness!

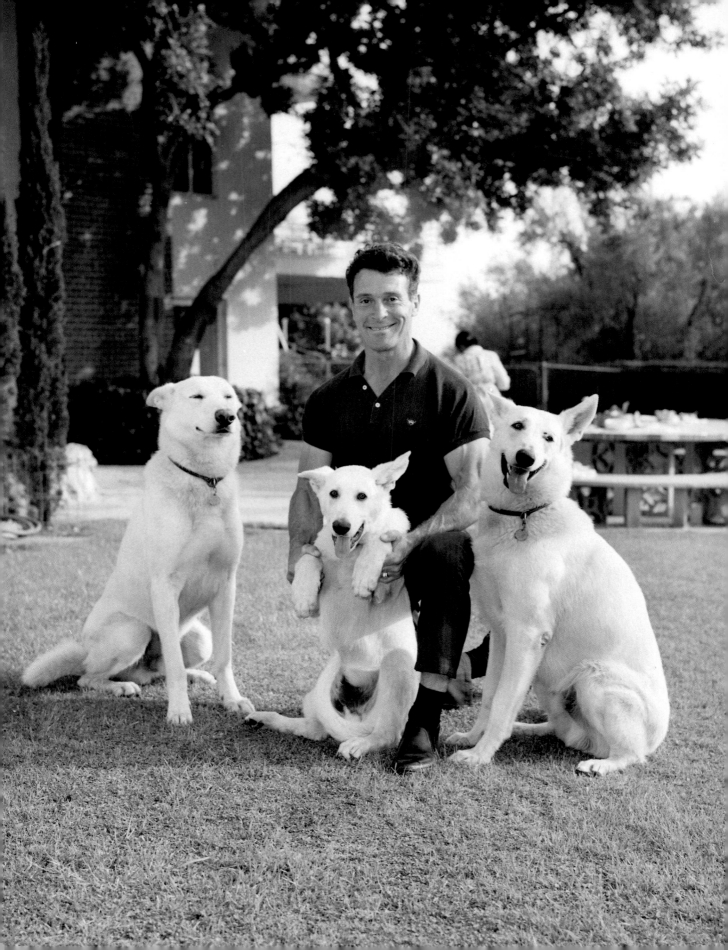

Of course today body odor is considered objectionable by most. If you want to win friends and influence people, shower regularly. And do more than just a quick wash of your body. Concentrate on the target areas. Use a deodorant soap on the groin and armpit. If you feel you have a heavy problem remember your perspiration glands work both night and day shifts. This means you might need a shower both morning and night.

HAIR CARE

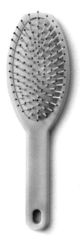

Hairdressers tell us dandruff is the single most common scalp complaint. Dermatologists tell us virtually everyone has the problem to some degree. It is important to shower and shampoo regularly. Don't ignore the condition or the flakiness will worsen. Use an antidandruff formula if regular shampooing doesn't work. When using the shampoo gently massage the scalp with your fingertips to help loosen the scales and flakes. Even those without a dandruff problem should wash their hair regularly. The root bed must be kept clean. Oil from the sebaceous glands, mixed with dirt and perspiration, can form a crust over the scalp and new hairs can't push through. Baldness is solicited.

Hair care starts with good nutrition. As men age they tend to lose hair where they want it and grow it where they don't, i.e. in their nose and ears. As a woman ages her hair tends to lose its luster and begins to thin. Excessive coloring and hair dryer use can damage the hair. Sweating and not washing can clog pores and cause hair loss. Curiously, sun, wind and freezing temperatures can thicken hair.

Brushing your hair with a natural bristle brush once a day for several minutes can help keep your hair lustrous and strong.

A good diet and exercise program will help your hair too, believe it or not. Anything bad for your body is bad for your hair. Conversely, anything good for your body is also good for your hair.

SKIN CARE

Your skin reveals not only the outer you, but also the inner you. If you want to feel younger, you've got to maintain younger looking skin. I was a mass of pimples and boils in my early teens. I had craters and mountains on my face and back that looked like a relief photo of the moon. My skin alone gave me enormously low self-esteem. Only when I discovered superior nutrition and regular strenuous exercise did my skin improve.

What's the skin? It's the biggest gland in the body, the structure that holds us all in place and protects tissues from injury. Our skin also acts to regulate our body temperature, and it has power to eliminate waste products from the body via sweat.

Pour nutrition in general and the eating of junk food shows in the skin. I can look at a person and pretty much tell you what kinds of foods they eat on a regular basis. Faulty elimination shows in the skin, as does excessive sunshine, lack of sleep, the smoking of cigarettes, abundant drinking and a stressful lifestyle.

A point about sunshine. In earlier days I believed the more time I spent in the sun the better. I strived for a year-round polished-mahogany tan. Living in California made this possible. I felt great. But in my 30s I changed my opinion radically. A good suntan does give a man or woman a fresh outdoorsy appearance, but excessive sunshine cures the skin like leather. You can take on the appearance of a raisin or prune. Not good. On the other hand,

Your skin reveals not only the outer you, but also the inner you.

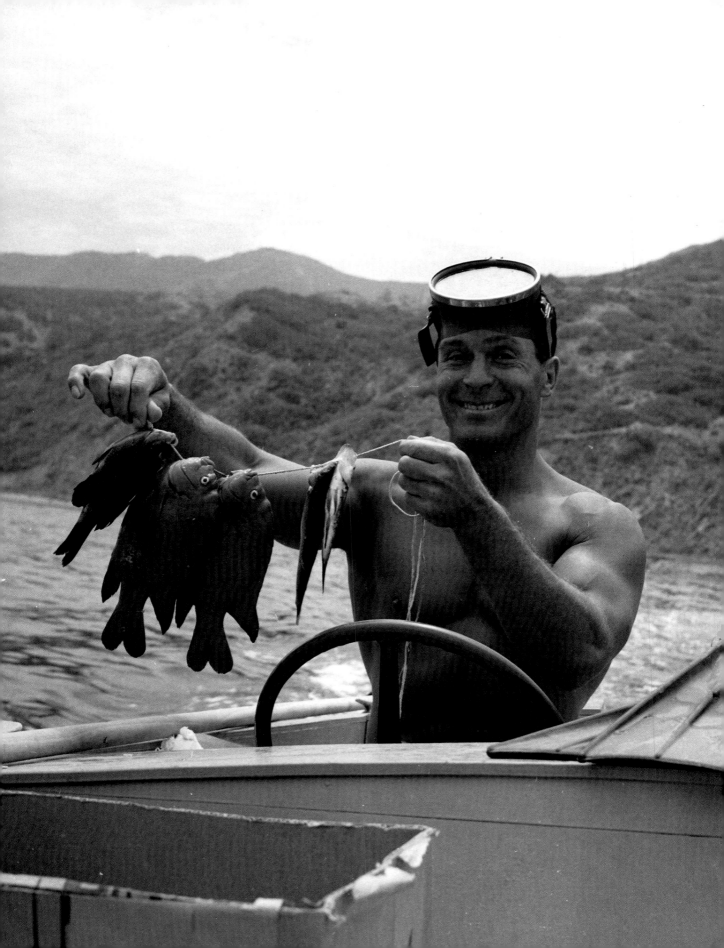

there would be no life on Earth without the sun, and a certain amount of sunlight is needed for health. Our fruits, grains and vegetables all harness the sun and absorb its rays, and nutritional goodness is amplified as a result. I'm sure you know by now that skin cancer caused by excessive sun can be lethal. Never allow your skin to burn in the sun. If you must face the sun (while cycling, boating, tennis, golf or a work project), then wear a hat and protective eyewear, and use protective sun lotion.

My position on tanning beds is negative. I do not feel they are healthy. Carolyn Ash, in her book *Timeless Skin* (Splash Publishing), calls them "cancer beds" and says: "Any exposure to the radiation from a tanning bed is too much." Unfortunately, some people feel impervious to the ill effects of tanning beds, even though they know they are dangerous. The only place you will find positive information on tanning beds is in brochures given out to promote their salons. I cannot give tanning beds my stamp of approval. There are numerous sunless tanning creams and lotions available, but bear in mind most sunless tanning lasts only two to three days after which you will need to reapply.

A good suntan does give you a fresh outdoorsy appearance, but excessive sunshine can cure your skin like leather.

TIPS ON KEEPING YOUR SKIN HEALTHY &
LOOKING GOOD

➜ Wash your skin thoroughly on a daily basis.

➜ Eat organic, natural foods when possible. Strive to reduce junk-food intake to zero.

➜ No tanning beds.

➜ No smoking.

➜ Turn that frown into a smile, now.

➜ Wash any new gym wear before using.

➜ Natural cotton products are superior to those containing polyester.

➜ If you are overweight you may want to put small amounts of petroleum jelly or talcum powder between your thighs, around your feet, in your underarms and around your nipples to avoid chafing when exercising.

➜ You don't have to buy expensive creams to get good results. Normal or dry skin reacts perfectly to lanolin, petroleum jelly, light mineral oil and cocoa butter.

➜ Women with oily skin should use only water-based cosmetics and light creams.

➜ Men with excessively oily skin should use an astringent after washing.

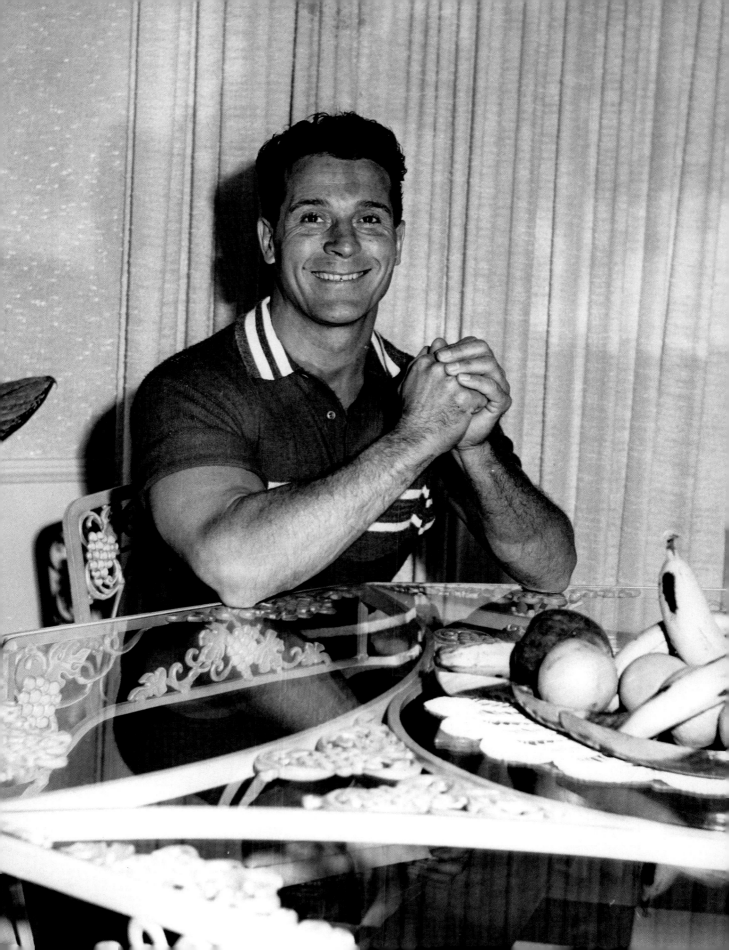

DENTAL CARE

I don't have one cavity in my mouth, but I had such a poor start it seemed I would be toothless by 25. As a sickly baby and, according to my mother, a constant crier, my mother cared for me while my father was at work. She couldn't stand my endless crying so, as I have related, she would fill a piece of cheesecloth with cornstarch and sugar and jam it into my mouth whenever I whimpered. This caused all my baby teeth to decay and turn black. My second teeth came in stained yellow. It was bad news. Nothing made my mother happier than when I started to eat wholesome foods. My mouth got a complete overhaul, and in no time I had a fresh looking mouth, free of cavities, all thanks to 100-percent improvement in nutrition. Taking care of your teeth is extremely important, because plaque and tartar buildup is not only damaging, it is downright obnoxious, unsightly and has an unpleasant odor.

Tartar buildup is damaging, obnoxious, unsightly and has an unpleasant odor.

Clean your teeth at least every morning and night. Keep a toothbrush at work so you can brush after eating lunch.

Flossing is more important than it may seem. Floss daily. It takes less than two minutes. Remember that tooth and gum problems can affect your heart adversely.

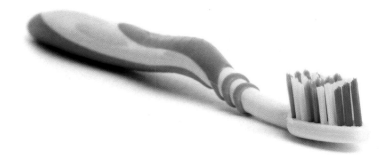

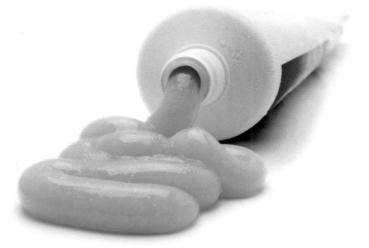

Your first duty, whether you have a dental problem or not, is to make an appointment with your dentist. Twice a year is good practice. Neglected teeth and tooth and gum decay can shorten your life. Periodontal disease (including gingivitis and periodontis) is due in large part to poor diet and poor dental hygiene. Miss out on brushing your teeth (especially at night, because the action of plaque is most damaging at night when the amount of tooth cleaning saliva in your mouth decreases) and you will have severe regrets in later years.

There is no proof that electric toothbrushes do a better job than manual brushing. However, if dexterity is a problem an electric brush will be the better tool. The back of your lower teeth is where plaque is most likely to hide. And don't be concerned with brushing only the smile surfaces; brush everywhere. According to expert Dr. William Campoli DMD, a Charlotte, NC dentist, "The areas where the teeth come into contact with the tongue and the cheek are where you need to concentrate your efforts.

Don't miss out on brushing your teeth (especially at night).

EYE CARE

What is it they say? Your eyes are the windows of your soul. Kinda true, huh? How often have you said to yourself, "I don't like the look in his eyes," or something similar? We read people by looking into their eyes. Have you ever gotten out of bed feeling okay with the world and yourself, but when you looked in the bathroom mirror and checked out your eyes, as we all do, you noticed by their appearance that you don't feel well at all. Yes, the eyes have the power to speak to us and let us know exactly how we feel.

Your eyes need exercise just like any other muscle, especially in this day of pollution, television, driving and computers. I am a great believer in exercising my eyes. Like a camera or a pair of binoculars when you adjust the focusing mechanism. I like to exercise my eyes by changing my focus on various objects. Maybe it's my restless nature. I can't sit still for long and I constantly want to look around me, observe and learn. Could be my French heritage, or is it the fact that I feel so energetic and good about myself I just want to explore? Anyways, I use this characteristic of mine to exercise my eyes. How do I do it? I grab a book with fine print (a telephone book will do, although with everyone owning a computer, I don't know how long the telephone company will continue to print books). Start by focusing on the small print, and then slowly bring the book up close to your face endeavoring to focus as it comes up to your nose. Oops! Now the Jones' and Smiths are really getting jumbled. Then, quick as a flash I look out of the window beyond Santa Monica, and try to focus on a sailboat way out near the horizon. Repeat this experiment

> I am a great believer in exercising my eyes.

several times a week. Look at objects up close and way out. And from distance again to up close. This practice has enabled me to see clearly without glasses since I was in my teens, at which time the only focusing I did was at the candy counter at the corner store. I believe focusing the eyes to be a very useful eye-strengthening exercise. However, the practice is only recommended for healthy eyes. If you have eye problems then your first course for action is to consult your eye doctor. He's the real professional, fully trained to treat abnormal eye conditions. I gave eye and face exercises on my TV show for years and I currently market a DVD specifically dedicated to the subject.

Name _____

Address _____

_____ Date _____

R͓X

If you have eye problems then your first course for action is to consult your eye doctor.

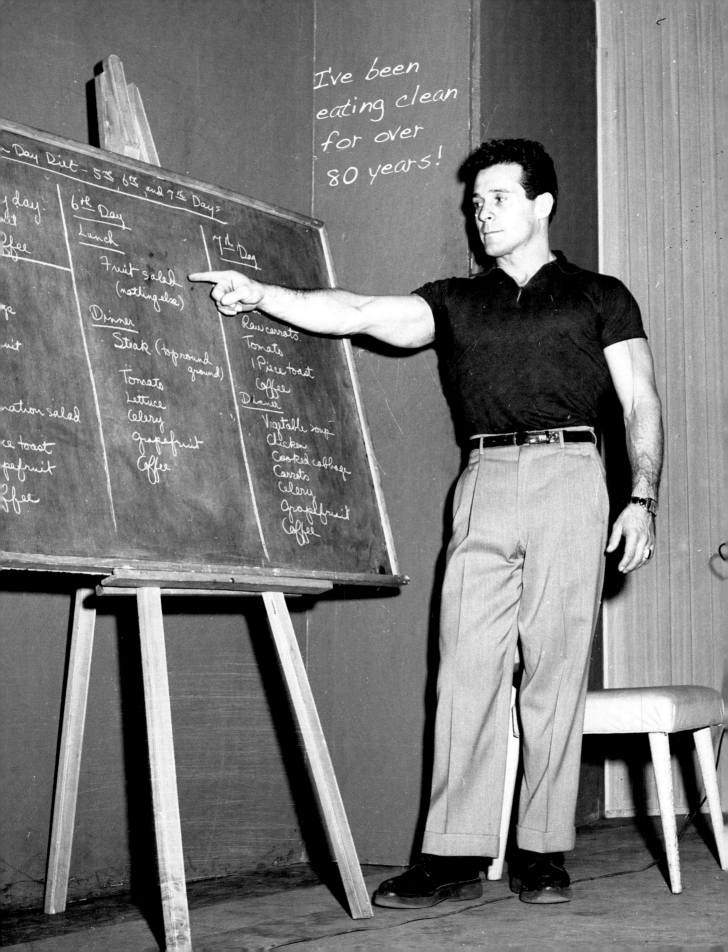

CHAPTER SEVEN

Step 4:
Eating Clean

TOMORROW IS WHAT YOU EAT TODAY.

Ever since my teens, when I first attended Paul Bragg's seminar in San Francisco, I have been eating only the most nutritious foods. In the health lecture I refer to earlier in this book, memories of this man were magnified by the fact that he singled out my mother and me when we arrived at his seminar. There was nowhere to sit, so we had started to leave when, from the stage, Paul asked the security guards to grab a couple of seats which were placed on stage next to him and in front of the entire audience. Little wonder his message was drilled into my head. He talked positively about how everyone could take immediate steps to change their lives for the better. He was against alcohol abuse and tobacco and encouraged everyone to get into the habit of eating only the most nutritious foods along with exercises such as calisthenics and hiking. That day, I listened and followed. In the coming years I studied *Gray's Anatomy*, went to Chiropractic college and opened my first physical culture studio in 1936. Later in life Paul and I became close friends.

I believe most foods that have been tampered with or manufactured by man, or even foods that have undergone man's attempt at improvement … are less than perfect. And, I hasten to say, these foods are in all likelihood bad for our long-term health. What am I talking about? I'm talking about food coloring, preservatives, thickeners, thinners, so-called taste enhancers and the zillion other chemicals thrown into the foods we are buying and ingesting every day, week after week, year after year. In addition to this catastrophic state of affairs we are also eating meat,

> I believe that most foods manufactured by man are less than perfect.

fish and poultry and produce that has been grown or raised on farms, most of which have been fed and dosed up with a variety of unnatural foods, hormones, antibiotics and chemicals. It doesn't take a genius to realize if we eat products that have been loaded up with poor-quality or even distinctly harmful foods or drugs, then those same ingredients will be passed down to our own bodies ... and we will suffer the consequences.

Now, let me ask you this: Do you or your significant other shop correctly? Do you regard it as a necessary evil, a chore? Is your mind elsewhere as you push the grocery cart between the aisles? Are you trying to remember your grocery list? Do you read labels? Are you at all concerned over whether or not the foods you pick are going to enhance your health and longevity – or are you just concerned with how the picture on the box appears, tasty or not so tasty? Are you stressed during your grocery shopping?

When my wife and I go shopping we enjoy the experience. Even today, I often remind myself of the goodness of the produce I buy. I look for crisp, green lettuce, hardy watermelon, fresh rasp-

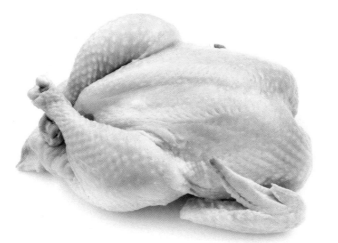

Poultry raised on farms are often fed and dosed up with unnatural hormones and chemicals.

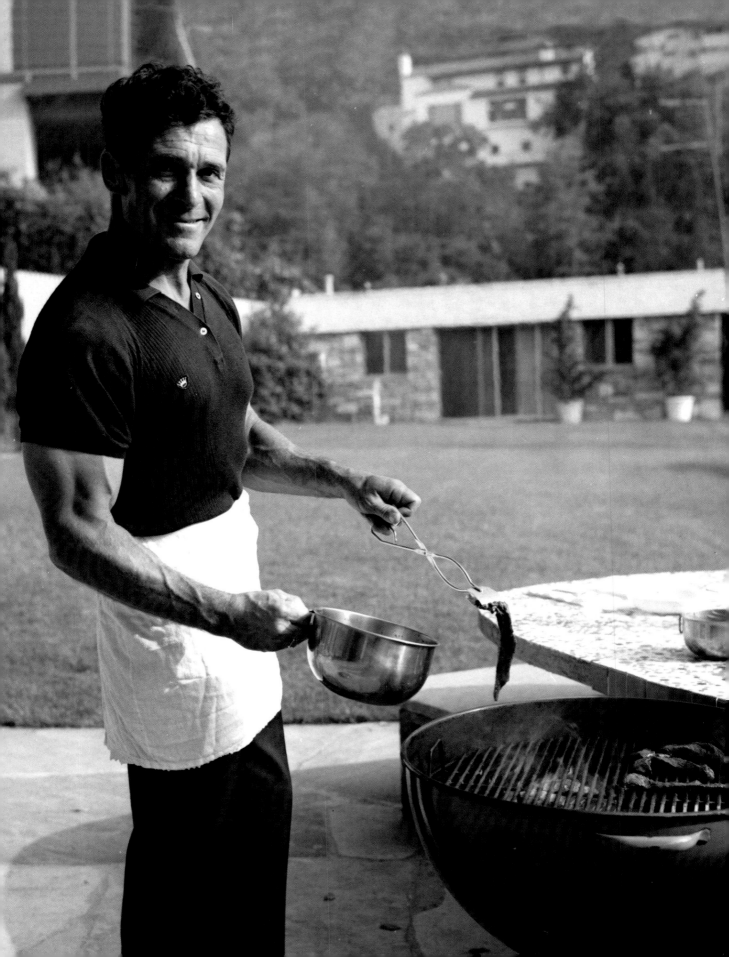

berries, oatmeal, Granny Smith apples, and brown rice. I read the labels of new products and give those sweet-smelling aisles that offer boxed gooey cakes and biscuits a complete miss. To go down them almost makes me want to throw up.

And talking of boxed products, I observed a guy in our local grocery store a couple of months ago. He looked totally confused. We got talking. It turned out he was on his first visit to the US, arriving only a day earlier from a small town in a third world country. Why was he confused? He had never seen boxed up or packaged food before! He told me everything in his village store was sold in its natural state, whether it be chicken, bread, fruit, rice, or what have you. Now he was staring at packaged cereals, biscuits, cakes and even plastic containers with cut up fruit slices or mixed salads. I'll never forget the bewildered look he had on his face. Of course, we North Americans are not the only ones to mess with the foods nature has given us; this is becoming a world-wide event. Right from my teens I've been in favor of eating foods as close to their natural state as possible. When man has had his hand in the manufacturing of a food, I simply say: no thank you.

In many ways we are lucky today. There is an abundance of farmers' markets, grocery and specialty stores that can deliver fine health-giving produce. But we simply have to shop intelligently. Make it a rule to always buy the freshest, most nourishing of mineral-rich foods. Buying cheap, packaged or adulterated foods or eating at fast-food establishments is not only bad for your health and longevity, it is poor economy. You may save a buck or two, but balance your expense against what you might have to spend on seltzers, laxatives, antacids or even doctors and you'll

Make it a rule to always buy the freshest, most nourishing of mineral-rich foods.

Prepackaged or fast food costs much more than natural food.

realize the error of your ways. Besides, if you honestly look at the price of all the food you eat, you will see prepackaged or fast food costs much more than natural food. And I firmly believe American families save by learning and practicing the basics of good nutrition. You can't be efficient in your daily work and in your family obligations unless you feed yourself with proper nutrition. Sending a pooped-out body off to work with a piece of toast and a cup of coffee is an invitation to failure.

You've heard it a thousand times: You are what you eat. In my seminars I'll sometimes tell the audience: What you eat today will be walking and talking tomorrow. Just as you put the best fuel in that hot new automobile, so should you feed your body only the very best. Food is what we use to build and repair our body tissue. The quality of your blood, brain and muscles will be in direct relation to the quality of the food you eat.

Think clearly before you enter your local grocery store. Determine before you enter you will buy only foods that will contribute to your health and that of your family. And while you're at it, look down the street from your supermarket. See the offices of doctors, dentists, druggists and medical clinics? Their bills run into thousands of dollars, and a large proportion of their customers are there not only because they have ignored the basic health principles of controlling alcohol and tobacco, but because they have chosen, through ignorance or indifference, to eat the junk foods that form 80 percent of supermarkets' merchandise.

There is an art to shopping. When you enter the grocery store you immediately circle to the fruits and vegetables, that lavish display of tomatoes, peppers, carrots, raw peas, spinach, romaine, celery, leeks, cucumbers, onions … wow! Just bringing these veggies to mind makes my mouth water! There's more: Now we come upon the fruits. Check out those juicy apples, oranges, bananas, grapes, and pears. And what about the blueberries, strawberries, blackberries and raspberries? More excitement for the palate. Always pick the brightest, freshest colors. Actually, fruits and veggies should be selected fresh every day, but I am a realist and I'm aware that daily grocery shopping isn't always an option.

If you are within reach of a store or stand that features organically grown produce (grown *without* sprays, fertilizers, pesticides or chemicals), by all means use them in preference to others. Ironically, and you have to shake your head at this, those fruits and veggies grown naturally, without chemicals, are more expensive. Go figure. Naturally it is wise to thoroughly wash all farm-grown produce (whether organically grown or not) before eating. While fruits and vegetables may all look the same to the untrained eye, they offer vastly different amounts of minerals and vitamins, and thus long-term health results.

STEP

4

Develop a strong sense of being a grocery store food critic.

BUYING FRUITS AND VEGGIES

Develop a strong sense of being a grocery store food critic. Choose fruits and veggies with attention to eye appeal, general appearance, firmness, ripeness and even smell. Okay, so don't grab every apple and orange and stick it to your nose. You know how to do these things subtlety. Holding an apple up close can allow you to check it for bruises, and still give you the heads up on its overall freshness value, as a good or bad buy. A large percentage of apples and other fruits are bruised. And berries are frequently past their freshness if not outright bad.

OTHER GOODIES

What else do we buy when at a grocery store or health food outlet? How about some raw almonds? They are full of calcium, iron, vitamin E and riboflavin. Or what about Brazil nuts, full of phosphorous, selenium and thiamin, or sunflower seeds, contain potassium, zinc, folate and niacin?

Moving on to the milk section: pop a quart or two of skim milk into your grocery cart. Have you noticed there are more varieties of milk than ever before? Today you can tailor your milk to your current allergy profile. There is whole milk, raw milk, milk with 1%, or 2% fat, milk high in calcium, milk that is lactose free; you name it. There is milk for everybody.

Getting to the breads and cereals, I like the whole-grain varieties. There are hosts of whole-grain wraps and brown-bread variations to suit your palette. Stay away from the white, devitalized breads and bagels. Check labels. You don't really want to have your cereals and breads full of salt and sugar, do you? Choosing

> One of my favorite foods is poached salmon.

a cereal? Go for muesli (a mixture of grains and nuts). Make sure there's no added salt or sugar.

I try to purchase only organically raised meat and fish. One of my favorite foods is poached salmon along with a salad of eight to ten chopped, raw vegetables. I like other types of fish as well – no batter of course, and served with steamed vegetables. If serving chicken, your best bet would be skinless chicken breast. Eggs are also a source of great nutrition. They possess the highest-quality protein available. I personally eat four to eight egg whites a day, usually hardboiled. Although whole eggs contain high cholesterol, they are also are high in iron. So if you don't have a cholesterol problem, you may want to eat the whole egg from time to time.

Soy, tofu, hemp protein and other vegetarian products can replace animal protein quite easily. "Meat" should not be the centerpiece of the meal; veggies are!

As we push our carts around the grocery store we begin to notice a certain sickly sweet smell invading our nostrils. Oh, no!

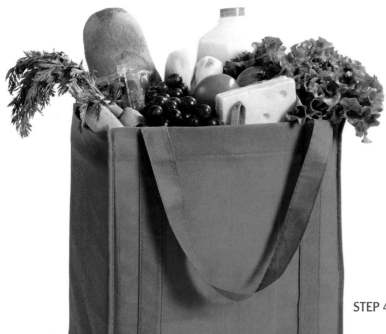

Choose fresh foods instead of canned as much as possible.

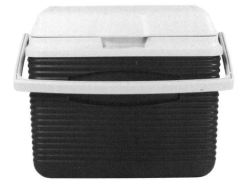

Pack a cooler. It's the smart thing to do.

We're approaching the cookies, cakes, biscuits and other sugar-loaded garbage foods. Hurry through this zone. Don't stop to check out even one item. Same goes for the pre-packaged and canned foods sections. You might pick up the odd item like a few cans of water-packed tuna for emergencies, but don't make a habit of eating out of cans. Choose fresh foods instead of canned as often as possible. The same goes for all those packaged TV dinners and other boxed-up food items. Stay away.

I am a calorie counter. No one knows how many calories they burn up each day and no one knows how many calories they are ingesting. By all means be aware of which foods are high and which are low in calories, and adjust your portions accordingly. You can do this by buying a calorie counter; it is a good way to manage your diet.

Once we have committed to eating only the most nourishing and healthy foods we have to watch out for the everyday traps that can sabotage our efforts. In the early days our First Nations peoples had to plan their eating by packing meals in advance of going on visits or traveling to other areas of the country. And in the modern day, in your own life — if you are planning on going for a sail, you will, no doubt, plan a lunch in advance. After all, there are no restaurants in the open water (at least not yet!). Why should things be any different when going to work, traveling in the car with family and friends, or going for a hike? You pack a cooler. It's the smart thing to do.

If your day is like those of most people, you spend time away from the house for a substantial part of the day, either at work or following through with some errands. If this is the case for you, whether every day or only on occasion, then during this time you will need to feed yourself. And often the only establishments around are fast-food enterprises or restaurants that have no concept of what constitutes good nutrition. So the sensible answer is pack a cooler. Load it with delicious, nutritious foods. Like what? Apples, chicken breast, raw veggies, celery, sprouts, almonds, bananas, whole-grain wraps, brown rice, unsweetened applesauce, water-packed tuna, grapes, berries, hot-cooked cereal, muesli, skimmed milk, low-fat plain yogurt, whole (hardboiled) eggs, and low-fat cheese. They are all good choices.

Packing a cooler may seem like hard work, especially in the beginning, but after you have got into the habit it will be second nature. And your healthy, fit, energetic beautiful physique will thank you for it.

You probably won't need a jumbo-sized cooler. Look for a soft-sided cooler just large enough to hold two or three small meals. When you buy your cooler, assuming you don't already have one, pick up a few re-freezable ice packs. Finally, don't forget to include some bottled water in your cooler. This doesn't have to be plastic bottles you purchase; rather, it can be refillable stainless or aluminum bottles.

When you buy your cooler, pick up a few re-freezable ice packs.

Now, what kind of foods are you ingesting? Are they live and vital or dead foods? Ask yourself "What are these foods going to do for me?" Did you know about every 60 to 90 days practically every cell in your body is replaced? So if you improve your eating and exercise habits, those new cells should be superior to the old ones. Right? Remember: "What you eat today is walking and talking tomorrow," and: "Ten seconds on the lips and a lifetime on the hips." Here are some sample menus to help you eat for health, fitness and longevity. Adjust your portions to fit your natural appetite.

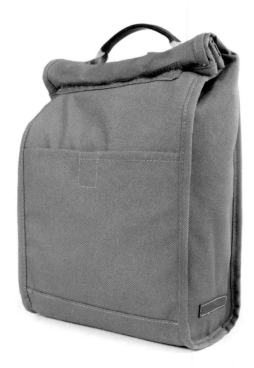

DAY ONE

BREAKFAST
→ Hot oatmeal and blueberries
→ Omelet made of 2-6 egg whites
→ 2 glasses of water
→ 1-2 slices whole-grain toast
→ Green tea or coffee

MID-MORNING
→ Orange
→ Glass of water

LUNCH
→ Grilled skinless chicken breast
→ Salad

MID-AFTERNOON
→ ½ cup almonds
→ Glass of water

SUPPER
→ Grilled salmon
→ Steamed veggies
→ Fresh fruit cup
→ Water

LATE-NIGHT SNACK
→ Granny Smith apple

DAY TWO

BREAKFAST

→ Oatmeal pancakes

→ 2 glasses of water

→ Mixed fruit cup

→ Coffee

MID-MORNING

→ Juiced fruit and veggies

LUNCH

→ Chili

→ 1-2 slices whole-grain bread

→ 1 cup of strawberries

MID-AFTERNOON

→ ½ cup almonds

SUPPER

→ Bison

→ Steamed veggies

→ Brown rice

LATE-NIGHT SNACK

→ ½ cup unsweetened applesauce

DAY THREE

BREAKFAST

→ Muesli with skim milk

→ Scrambled egg whites with tomatoes

→ 1-2 glasses of water

→ Green tea

MID-MORNING

→ 1 cup cottage cheese

LUNCH

→ Homemade meat and veggie soup

→ 1-2 slices whole-wheat bread

→ 1-2 glasses of water

MID-AFTERNOON

→ Fat-free plain yogurt

SUPPER

→ Grilled sea bass

→ Sweet potato

→ Mixed salad

→ ½ cup berries

LATE-NIGHT SNACK

→ ½ banana

DINING OUT
DOING IT RIGHT

People who know me as a person into healthy nutrition are surprised to discover that Elaine and I eat out every night of the week except Monday, when we usually have a few friends over to watch Monday Night Football or whatever sport is featured that evening. I have to admit that when we go out for our evening meal, we are spoiled. Our favorite restaurants know exactly what we want. In fact, the main dish at each establishment is invariably known as the Jack LaLanne Special.

Why do we eat out? Because we work hard at giving seminars and interviews, promoting the Jack LaLanne Juicer, and even writing books and attending book signings. We've given some 70-plus years to earning a living while helping others to reach for a new healthy lifestyle, and we like to be waited on now and again. Eat-

My wife Elaine and I had to learn how to eat right while on the road giving seminars.

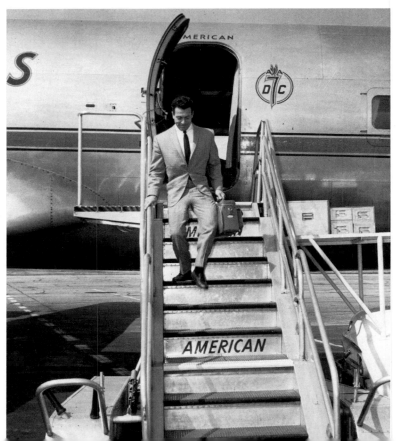

ing in a fine restaurant is a social outing for us. We patronize several restaurants in our area, and the servers and chefs know exactly how we like our fish and steamed veggies followed by a dessert of fresh berries. Dining out is a luxury for us even today. We enjoy people, and it's fun, especially since now in California and most other states, smoking is not allowed in public places.

Dining at a restaurant is only a problem if you allow it to be so. Admittedly some restaurants are better than others, but in 80 percent of food-providing establishments you will be able to find acceptable nourishment that will not contribute to fat accumulation or ill health.

Step one: Make friends with your server. Give him or her a warm smile and explain with gentleness that you want your fish without sauce, the vegetables have to be steamed, no butter added. Take your baked potato without butter or sour cream. No dressing on the salad. Balsamic vinegar and extra virgin olive oil is the healthy choice. When you have soup it has to be broth based as opposed to cream based. No butter or cream. Personally, I love soup. Gravy is a no-no. Want a dessert? How about berries or a fresh fruit salad?

Breakfasting out? Go for hot oatmeal (no sugar-loaded cereals), with fresh berries. Make sure it's made with water, not milk. Follow that with a vegetarian egg-white omelet and ask that it be cooked in a little olive oil, not canola, corn oil or butter. A slice or two of whole-grain toast without butter rounds off the meal. I'm personally not into coffee, but a cup or two a day isn't sinfully bad. Forget the cream and sugar, of course. I prefer to choose from the large variety of herbal teas available today.

STEP
4

Dining at a restaurant is only a problem if you allow it to be so.

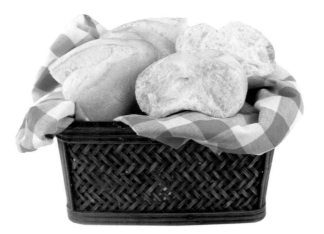

Many restaurant eaters make the mistake of loading up on bread before the meal even begins.

Many restaurant eaters make the mistake of loading up on bread before the meal even begins. Worse, they add butter. Then they have two or three cocktails and nibble on other goodies. They overeat at the beginning and then are satiated prior to the main course and hardly enjoy the outing. If you really want an appetizer, ask for some raw veggies without the dip.

Restaurants are potential traps that can easily sabotage your fitness goals. Because Elaine and I eat out virtually every night, we learned years ago to enjoy the experience. We always maintain control of what we consume. I'm smiling as I write this because I know how easy it is for everything to go wrong. I have dined with friends who let the waiter take control. It's as though they give in to temptation "just this once."

The other day a friend of mine and I were eating lunch after a business meeting. He asked the waiter if the soup of the day was cream or broth based. "It's cream based, sir," came the reply. "Oh, I can't eat that," said my friend, "I need a broth-based soup. I'm watching my calories."

"Too bad," smiled the waiter. "It's very tasty; our customers love it!"

"Okay," replied my friend. "Give me a bowl, just this once."

Before you go into a restaurant I want you to stop at the entrance and make a promise to yourself not to weaken when you see the menu or hear the waiter talk about the restaurant specials.

A frequent occurrence at restaurants is the failure of the chef to listen to the waiter's request. Salads have a fat- and calorie-dense dressing poured over them. The egg-white omelet has cheese in it (most cheese is more than 50 percent fat, by calories). A dollop of cream has been arranged prettily in the middle of your soup bowl. The whole-grain toast has butter on it. Your baked potato is covered in sour cream.

So what do you do? I'll tell you what 80 percent of diners do. They accept it and chow down! What you *should* do is pick up the plate and hand it back to the waiter, reminding him of what you actually ordered. This is always a nuisance because it causes a delay in you getting your original order, but it *has* to be done.

Restaurants often skimp on their salads, opting for a wedge of lettuce with the odd tomato slice. I ask the waiter to tell the chef to cut up some of the vegetables he has back there in the kitchen. A little balsamic vinegar can improve the experience, and voila! We have a tasty and healthy salad.

An old acquaintance of mine who ran several Jack LaLanne Health Clubs, Harry Schwarz, now retired, exercises and eats clean all the time. Recently he was dining with a group of former business friends. He politely asked for his fish to have no butter

A frequent occurrence at restaurants is the failure of the chef to listen to the waiter's request.

or sauce, for the vegetables to be steamed and the baked potato to have no butter or sour cream attached.

"No problem," said the server as he took down the order. You can guess what happened. It was as though the server had not heard a word. Or at least he failed to communicate the instructions effectively to the chef. When the meal arrived the server gracefully placed the plate in front of Harry, blissfully unaware that the fish was covered in a creamy white sauce and the baked potato was smothered with the biggest dollop of sour cream imaginable. Harry held his anger in check but was firm in his complaint, making no bones about his disappointment. "I made my wishes very clear to you," he said. "You apparently wrote everything down. And when I emphasized the importance of getting the order right, you told me 'No problem.' Well, we now have a problem, don't we?" He sent the meal back and had to wait a further 20 minutes to get what he had ordered in the first place. Harry apologized to his friends, who probably thought he was super picky. But his commitment to clean eating is why he is one of the healthiest octogenarians in America. We've all been through similar circumstances. Just make sure you don't cave and say, "Okay, leave it. I'll eat it as is. Just this once." If you have to pay for that meal your normal tip should be nonexistent or drastically reduced. If the

Make a promise to yourself not to weaken when you see the menu.

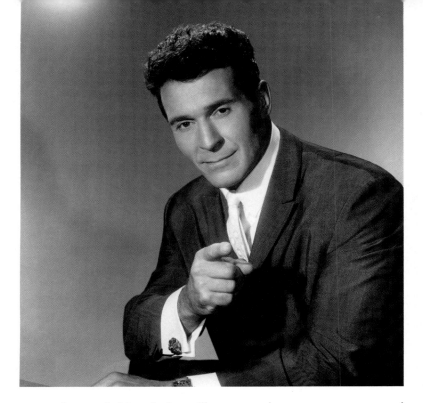

server is worth his salt, he will arrange that you get your meal free or at half price.

Now let's go out to a dinner party where the hosts pride themselves on the elegance of their cuisine. Whereas no one can force you to eat something you don't want, you will have to exercise a little caution in your approach. A good host won't insist you eat a food when you decline politely. The problem is being too unbending or forceful in your refusal can make the host uncomfortable and even give the other guests the feeling they are doing something wrong. If you feel you can't mention you are being careful in your diet, pass on something you don't want and eat more of what you do. Or simply take very small portions. Avoid the gravies and dressings on the table. Remove the skin from the fish or chicken. Should your host insist you try her favorite dessert, take the smallest portion and let most of it remain on your plate. Above all be polite but don't give in to sabotage, whether deliberate or innocent.

A good host won't insist you eat a food when you decline politely.

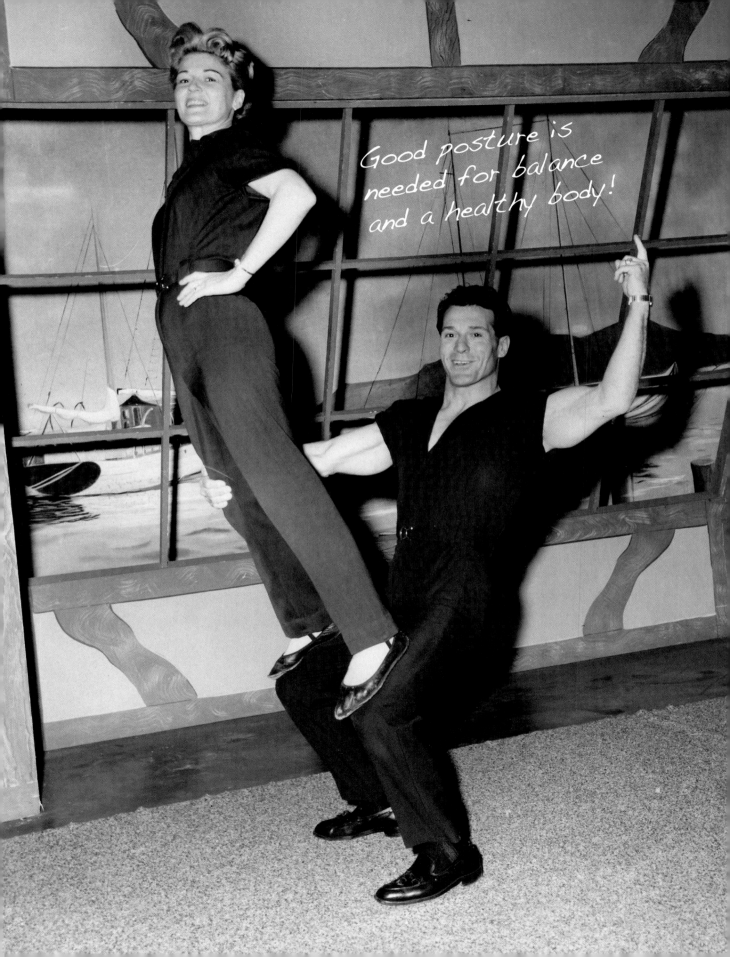

Good posture is needed for balance and a healthy body!

Step 5: Maintain Perfect Posture

COUNTENANCE COUNTS

The reason I am writing this book, at 95 years of age, is simple. I want you to come alive again. I want you to enjoy every minute of life. I want you to bloom. One of the aims of this book is to get you to revisit the body of your youth. With the nutritional and exercise advice I give you on these pages, I have no doubt that we can achieve that goal. When I pass on to that great gym in the sky I want no more than for people to say: "He was marvelously alive!" And I want the same for you.

The next time you are around a crowd of people, take a long hard look. Notice how really impressive figures are few and far between. Check out the appalling posture of the average school-aged kid. It's depressing. They stoop because they want to be accepted among their friends. They don't want to seem cocky, snooty or holier than thou. Pleas from parents or teachers to stand up straight are ignored and as the years roll into the late teens and early 20s, the poor posture is "set" and all but irreversible. It's sad, because a strong erect posture expresses to the world at large strength of will, alertness, poise and joy of living.

Always sit and stand with your back straight, stomach in and head up. Walk in the same way. When you come across a mirror, turn sideways and quickly reset your stance to reflect a perfect countenance. It will pay off.

My friend, octogenarian Bob Delmonteque, is 6 feet 3 and still has great posture. He's worked for it. At 65 Bob was financially stable from being an owner/operator of over 500 health clubs, but on retiring he started to relax his normally alert and active body. He got into the couch. He got into the beer. Then a

Always sit and stand with your back straight.

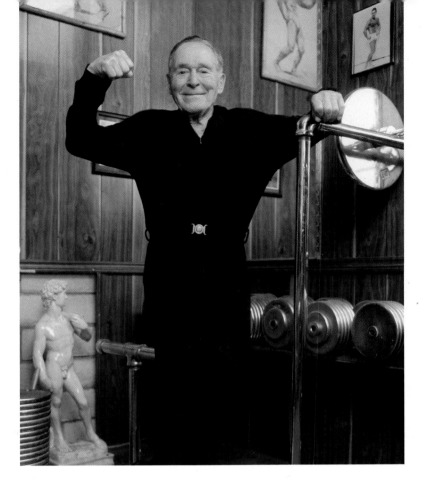

wakeup call came. Truth to tell, Bob had been a physical culturist since his teens and had made his fortune working hard as a personal trainer and in the aforementioned gym business. Bob confided in his friend Dr. Tony Quinn: "I think I'm going downhill." The two of them got together and made a plan. The conclusion was: "We must grow younger, not older." My sentiments exactly. Bob and the good doctor had come to the same conclusion I had many years earlier.

"We must
grow younger,
not older."

One of the first steps Bob took, after realizing that to grow old is a decision, was too improve his way of standing, walking, sitting. He worked on his posture and almost immediately started looking and feeling healthier. Then he regained his interest in exercise and good nutrition. He was on the mend and on his way to the superior health and strength he enjoys today.

Correct posture helps control stress, and also keeps us healthy and active. Poor posture can cramp the internal organs and causes numerous aches and pains as we get older. This affects our mobility.

As we age our neck begins to move forward, causing our back to slouch and slump. As you can imagine, when one part of the body is out of alignment the other areas are also offset. The domino effect is taking hold. One thing people sometimes don't understand is that their body will grow to the shape and posture they adopt. Typical of this is the evidence offered by the long-distance cyclist who spends hours in the hunched-over position on his bike. His back becomes irreversibly hunched. The more you slump, the more you lose flexibility so you not only move older, you feel older and you appear older.

Good posture is needed for proper balance and is a prerequisite for a healthy body. Also, the person who carries him or herself with a proud upright posture is more likely to come across as a fit, energetic, desirable individual. Yes, you are more attractive.

Correct posture helps control stress, and also keeps us healthy and active.

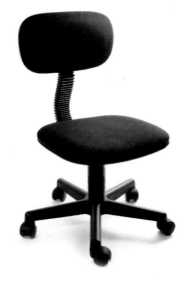

Good posture isn't just a matter of keeping your back straight and tummy in. You need to hold your shoulders back and your head up. Too, your shoulders and pelvis should be horizontal, not tilted to one side. Your arms should hang relaxed and your hands and fingertips should be level.

You should make a habit of checking your posture and correcting it if necessary. The worst type of stance to my mind is what I call *the lazy posture*. It belongs to the young. It's carefree, and downright ugly, and frequently becomes even uglier when linked with the inevitable dangling cigarette. If lazy posture is not corrected it becomes your permanent posture; and ugly is the only word for it. Besides, the by-product of ill posture is ill health … along with a lifetime of pain.

Check points: Do I stick my buttocks out too obviously, thus causing a swayback appearance? Are my shoulders slumped forward, causing my scapulae to stand out like wings in my back? Am I balancing evenly on my feet, not bearing my weight entirely on my heels? Do I round my back and slump forward at the table while eating my soup? Do I tilt my head permanently to one side while writing or using the computer? Do I allow my head to stick out in front of my body?

The beauty about deportment is that it doesn't have to make you look older − it can make you look younger. I believe that posture can reveal as much about you as your face does. Poor posture can make you a walking billboard of insecurity and old age. People who are tired often have poor posture, so you had better make sure you are getting your proper allocation of sleep and rest. Whether you are sitting or standing you are always fight-

I believe that posture can reveal as much about you as your face does.

ing gravity. (What else could make your ears double their length by the time you hit your 80s?)

When you are fighting gravity, everything tends to drop. Your face, neck, ears, shoulders and chest all want to drop. Ever see those old country homes, so old that they are sinking into the ground? What about that old car left to rust in the desert? Gravity takes it down, down, down. The coal found in mines miles below the earth's surface was once a blossoming, healthy tree. What took it to the depths of the Earth? Gravity! It's tugging at you and me this very moment. Let's fight back and prevent our youthful posture from wandering off.

Remember that attraction is the greatest factor in love. It's hard to relate easily to a man or woman you find unattractive. We all enjoy relating to attractive people. And posture is a key ingredient in attractiveness. A man who has an obese body with a bloated belly will likely look too unathletic to interest his loving wife. Similarly, a man may find it impossible to respond amorously to his wife if she looks unkempt, dowdy, obese and gives the distinct impression of not caring about her health, hygiene or appearance. The key here is sex appeal.

That's the point I'm trying to make. Posture is the one thing we can all improve instantly. And then in time we can make other significant changes. Good posture doesn't just make us look younger, slimmer and more attractive. Bad posture can wreck your health. Bad posture can be the cause of trouble with women's reproductive organs, and can also lead to faulty elimination as we age. Even your heart and lungs can be pushed around by repeated slouching posture, causing difficulty in getting sufficient

Posture is a key ingredient in attractiveness.

oxygen to the necessary vital functions. Poor posture can – and often does – lead to lower-back problems.

Ever see a group of marines marching? Now there's a sight. The way they carry their bodies, the set of their shoulders. Their deportment is 100 percent ideal. Is there any doubt about the health and vitality of these marching superhumans?

How can we improve our posture at this late date? One: Quit overeating, overdrinking and smoking. Two: Start exercising regularly three or four times a week. Three: Check and correct your posture throughout the day.

Have I convinced you with my preamble about the important of good posture? I really hope so. It is important and the effects are far-reaching. When you walk, walk as if you were seven feet tall.

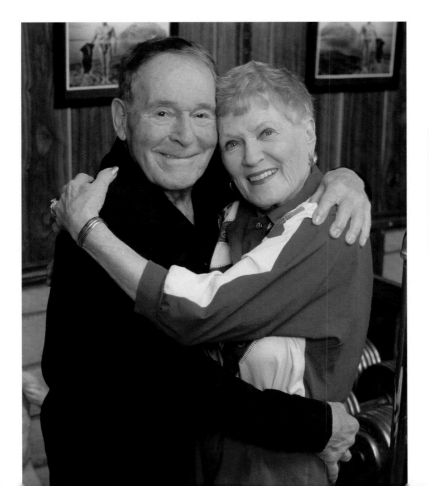

Remember that attraction is the greatest factor in love.

115

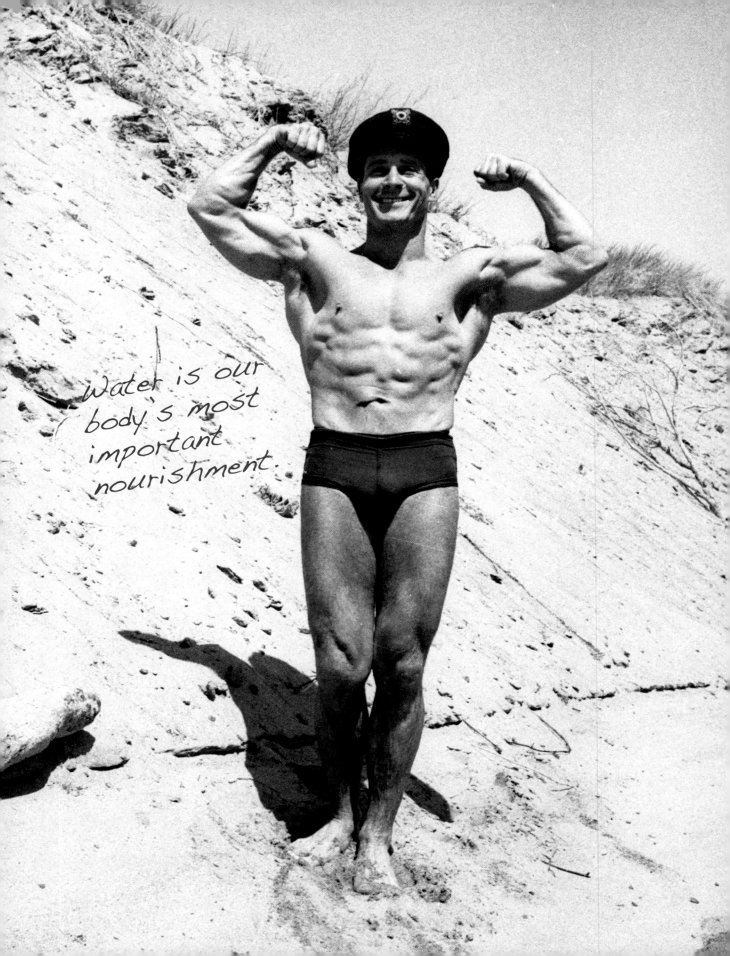

Water is our body's most important nourishment.

CHAPTER NINE

Step 6: Stay Well Hydrated

YOUR BODY IS THIRSTING FOR WATER.

Even today I pinch my solid biceps and wonder, 'Can I really be 70 percent water?' Ah, but scientists assure us it is so. Besides, we learned that in biology class, no? Anyway, as hard as my muscles look and feel, it is true: over two-thirds of our bodyweight is water. There's no doubt that water, the forgotten nutrient, is our body's most important nourishment. Lack of water can play havoc with your body, however balanced your diet.

Americans have for some time enjoyed a love affair with fizz. Witness the vast array of sodas, spritzers, champagne, colas and other fizzy drinks that are available to the buying public. Of course all these products contain water, as do your fruit and veggies – even a baked potato is 70 percent water – but I want you to get your hydration not from these options, nor from coffee, tea or beer, but rather from pure natural mineral water. How much? Two quarts a day!

Americans have enjoyed a love affair with fizz, but I want you to get your hydration from pure natural mineral watrer.

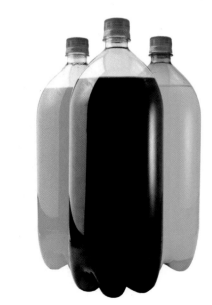

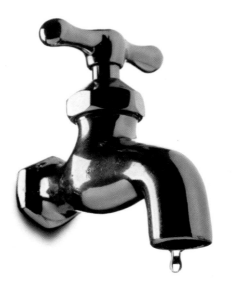

Why? 'Cos pure water is crucial to your health and appearance. For example, your skin, the body's largest organ, is a huge reservoir of water, but is the last to benefit from the water you consume. So if you are not getting your share, your skin will suffer. Water is found in the inner layer (dermis) of skin. While older people may not feel thirst the way they did in their younger years, they definitely need to keep their water intake high. Our skin tends to dry out naturally when we are older. If you're not drinking two quarts daily, then begin today. A couple of glasses in the morning is a good start.

How healthy is tap water? Are we not told time and time again that bottled water, even the most expensive, is no better than tap water? My answer to that is: Depends on the country and state. Some water is good; some not so good. Since you are going to be drinking two quarts of water a day, unfiltered tap water isn't your healthiest option. News items often report contaminated water reservoirs, rivers, and water-processing plants all over North America.

What goes hand in hand with efficient water consumption is the eating of fresh fruits and vegetables. For example, romaine lettuce, tomatoes, watercress and zucchini all contain over 95 percent water. And virtually all other fruits and veggies are made up of 85 percent water. The least thirst-quenching food is popped popcorn, at under 5 percent.

We use up water at an alarming rate. Even on a cool day if you are staying still your body uses 1 1/2 quarts of water. Most is excreted through the skin and kidneys and with every exhalation of breath (just breathe onto a mirror). And on blazing hot summer days we can only guess how much water we need. Add physical activity and the stupidity of alcohol consumption at such time, and we have a potentially very dangerous situation.

Water is also needed for elimination. It is vital that we eliminate our waste quickly. Constipation is the cause of many serious health problems. We never seem to get at the root causes of constipation. The principal reasons are lack of sufficient water and lack of exercise. Americans spend nearly two billion dollars annually trying to move their constipated bowels. My friend and mentor, the late Paul Bragg, claimed: "The chief reason we need so much bowel 'dynamite' is that we eat too much refined, mushy, lifeless, sugar-loaded unnatural foods." His remedy? You've guessed it: more fiber in the diet, regular exercise and plenty of water throughout the day. Paul Bragg also claimed that one bowel movement a day is not sufficient. He said, "No food should stay in the colon longer than 36 hours. People who have only one bowel movement a day are chronically constipated and carry 5 to 10 pounds of putrefying, fermenting food material in their lower bowel."

"No food should stay in the colon longer than 36 hours."

Foremost expert in the field of sports medicine Dr. Larry Perry says: "Even simply the act of breathing causes us to use approximately one pint of water each day. Our lungs need to be moistened by water to facilitate the intake of oxygen and the excretion of carbon dioxide."

When we don't drink enough water we tend to gain body-fat, because water helps with our digestion and metabolism. Most people haven't a clue as to how much water they should be drinking. In fact many older people are in a constant state of dehydration. A Johns Hopkins Medical letter (March 1993) stated, "Water is vital to every aspect of your body's physiological function. You need to keep your body in water balance."

Drink plenty of water to keep your body functioning properly and to wash all the toxins and impurities out of your system.

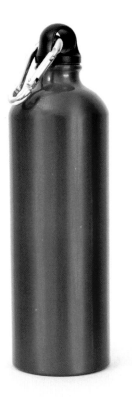

Drink plenty of water to keep your body functioning properly.

DO's AND DON'Ts OF
WATER DRINKING

✔ Do drink a natural mineral water whenever possible. Mineral water helps you make up vital minerals you lose throughout the day, especially during exercise, and doesn't contain additives. This water must come from an untainted source.

✔ Read labels: Look for the words natural mineral water or natural spring water. No, I'm not endorsed by them. Avoid products that say high sodium or high nitrates; both are capable of permanently damaging your body.

✔ Filter your tap water. Reverse osmosis or point-of-entry ceramic filters are the best. Both counter bacteria, viruses and other impurities.

✔ Do make a commitment to drink plenty of water if you are pregnant – more than eight glasses a day.

✔ Do limit the amount of caffeinated drinks you consume. For every caffeine-loaded soda (even diet cola), coffee, fizzy drink or tea you drink, you need to add one glass of water to your daily intake. Caffeine is a diuretic. Ditto with alcohol, also a diuretic.

✘ Don't gulp loads of cold water on a hot day or after strenuous physical exercise. Sip it slowly, preferably without ice.

✘ Don't fall for the misconception that avoiding water will dehydrate you and help you lose weight. If you are trying to lose weight, then it's fat you want to lose – not water. Our bodies must always be in correct water balance. Bringing yourself to dehydration is dangerous.

✘ Don't pay additional money for bottles labeled "table water." They can literally come from the same place as the water you pour out of your kitchen tap.

✘ As a general rule, stay away from fizzy drinks. Natural sparkling waters are acceptable but when artificial fizz is injected, minerals could be depleted.

✘ Distilled water is lacking some health components as it contains none of the minerals needed to enhance your healthy lifestyle.

✘ Regarding plastic containers. Most of us have been doing this for years, but modern research indicates that the practice is potentially unhealthy.

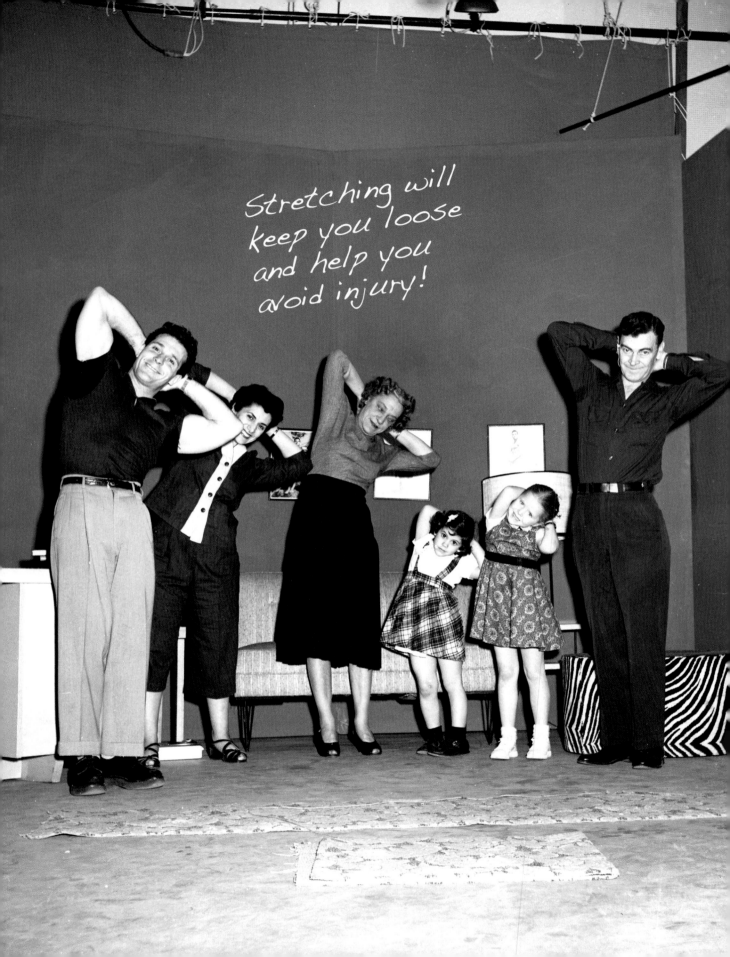

CHAPTER TEN

Step 7:
Stretching

EXTEND YOUR HORIZONS

It's surprising how many people are into health, strength and fitness but don't stretch. This is particularly true of those gym members known as bodybuilders. The first exercise they do upon entering the gym is the bench press, but do you think for one minute they are going to spend 10 minutes stretching their muscles before getting down and dirty with the weights?

Ever watch a cat stretch? Instinctively they feel the stretch, test the tension, focus on the stretch and then relax. You too? Stretching is important. I always make it part of my workouts and have been doing so for almost 80 years. Why stretch? It warms up your muscles, preparing you for the workout to come. It also increases your range of motion. Above all stretching keeps you limber and flexible, two joys of life we tend to ignore until we suffer the consequences of no longer having them. Stretching also helps us keep any injuries to a minimum.

Stretching warms up your muscles, preparing you for the workout to come.

Every workout should begin with a warm-up and stretching routine. Your weight or freehand exercises are important for your strength and stamina development, but the flexibility that comes with just 10 minutes of stretching on your workout days is priceless. It's your key to long-term independence and coordination.

The American College of Sports Medicine's statement on minimum fitness includes the requirement of regular stretching. We can begin to lose our flexibility from the very earliest years of childhood. Stiffness can begin to take hold as early as our 30s, and will progressively worsen with each successive year unless we challenge the barriers of flexibility on a regular basis. We all have limitations of flexibility and I'm not suggesting we aim for the range of motion associated with Cirque du Soleil performers, but don't disregard the added conditioning, good health and feeling of satisfaction that comes with flexibility and improved overall range of motion.

As 85-year-old Dr. Bob Delmonteque states in his popular seminars: "Tight joints and muscles are typically the result of inactivity – you lose the motions you do not use. Stretching loosens this tightness, lubricating the joints and allowing you to train each muscle through its complete range of motion."

Tight joints and muscles are typically the result of inactivity.

I always encouraged my TV crew to stretch often. It feels great!

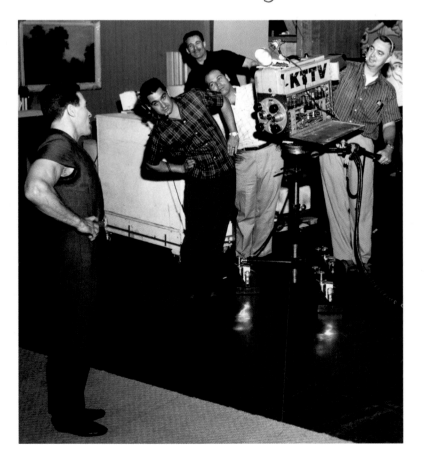

As we age we have the tendency to lose muscle, lose strength, lose flexibility, lose bone mass, lose sex drive, lose cardiovascular fitness, lose balance and generally lose our overall physicality. The good news is that we can grab our aging life by the shoulders and give it a good shake. We can refuse to let age run its plan of plummeting decline. Advancing years do not automatically spell future adversity or even limited enjoyment of all things physical. Osteoporosis and its associated problems are not inevitable.

WHEN YOU STRETCH REGULARLY YOU WILL:

➡ Warm up your muscles

➡ Increase flexibility and balance

➡ Reduce muscular tension

➡ Prepare yourself for exercise

➡ Increase the pleasure you get from everyday tasks

➡ Improve your circulation

➡ Increase coordination and agility

➡ Strengthen tendons, ligaments and muscles

➡ Improve your range of motion

➡ Enjoy occupations normally associated with youth

➡ Feel confident in the knowledge that you are supple, lithe and limber.

HOW TO BEGIN STRETCHING

Before commencing your weight training or other type of work-out, make a point of warming up your body. You should warm up before you begin stretching. This is simply a matter of hyping your circulation. Frequently we head off to the gym when we're not feeling 100 percent ready. We are lethargic and feel a little lazy, tired even. But this is easy to change! All we need to do is get up off the couch and walk. Speed it up; swing those arms. Get on the treadmill or stepper if you like, and get that heart pumping. Once you've got your blood pumping quickly through your arteries and veins, you'll start to feel warmer and more energetic. Now you actually feel like exercising. This is the best time to stretch!

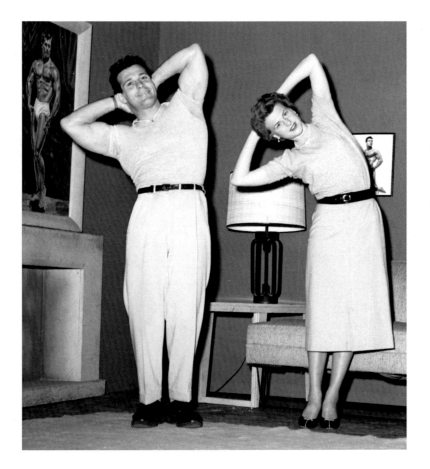

Get up off the couch and get your circulation moving!

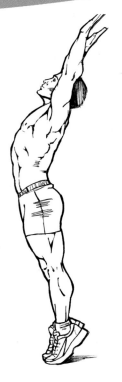

THE CEILING STRETCH

Stand with your feet shoulder-width apart. Lift your arms over your head, palms up; stretch as if you were trying to touch the ceiling or the sky. Count to 10, relax, then stretch, counting to 10 again.

SIDE-TO-SIDE STRETCH

Begin just as you would the Ceiling Stretch. While reaching for the ceiling, keep your feet planted solidly on the floor. Now, slowly and smoothly, bend at the waist from one side to the other. Count to 10 on each side. Relax and count to 10 again. Do not overstretch and do not use jerky movements.

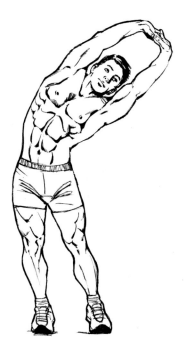

THROUGH THE LEGS STRETCH

Plant your feet shoulder-width apart. Bend forward at the waist, knees slightly bent to take the strain off the back. Bring the hands through the legs, attempting to touch the floor and wall behind you. Hold for a count of 10, relax, repeat and hold for a count of 10.

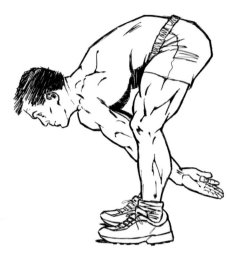

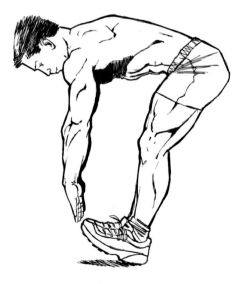

HAMSTRING STRETCH

Place your feet shoulder-width apart. Bend forward at the waist, knees bent very slightly. Allow your hands to drop down in front of your feet, as though trying to touch the floor. Now lift your toes off the floor. Hold for a count of five. Feel those hamstrings stretch.

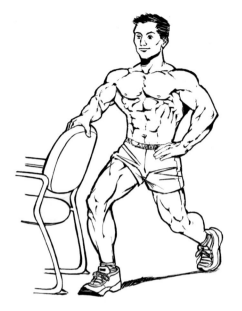

LEG LUNGE STRETCH

Stand erect, hands on hips (or on a chair for balance). Lunge forward (similar to a fencing pose). Hold for a count of five. Step back and lunge forward on the opposite leg and hold for a count of five. These can be done lunging to the side as well.

TIGER STRETCH

Stand with your hands clasped loosely behind your back and your feet shoulder width apart. Extend the clasped hands to arm's length behind you. Now try to touch your shoulder blades together and attempt to reach the wall behind you with your clasped hands. While doing this, elevate your head so you are looking at the ceiling. Feel your shoulders, stomach and hip muscles tighten? Now bend over at the waist, with knees bent, and look between your legs, hands still clasped at arm's length.

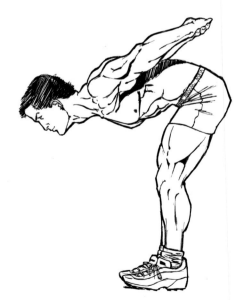

SHOULDER STRETCH

Stand with your knees slightly bent and your feet shoulder-width apart. Extend your left arm straight out. With your right hand, reach out and grasp your left elbow. Keeping the rest of your body – particularly your hips and shoulders – motionless, pull your left arm across your body toward your right shoulder as far as you can. Feel the stretch as you hold for five to ten seconds, then relax and repeat. Switch arms and repeat the exercise with your right arm.

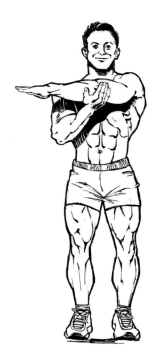

SEATED HAMSTRING STRETCH

Sit on the floor with your legs together and straight (or with one leg bent at the knee). With your arms straight, reach toward or past your toes, or bring your torso as close to your feet as you can.

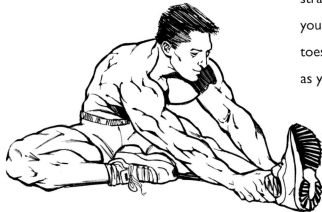

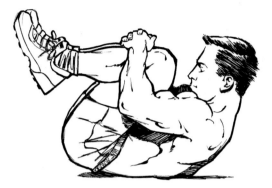

BACK STRETCH

Lie flat on the floor. Bend your knees, and place your hands around them. Pull your knees toward your upper chest while lifting your upper back off the floor.

QUADRICEPS STRETCH

Stand next to a wall or sturdy machine with your knees slightly bent and your legs shoulder-width apart. Tilt your hips forward slightly. With your right hand, brace yourself against the wall or machine. Lift your left leg behind you, curling it up so your foot approaches your glutes. Grasp your left foot in your left hand and slowly pull your foot toward your glutes. Feel the stretch as you hold for five to ten seconds. Return your left leg to the starting position, rest, and repeat. Then brace yourself with your left arm, and repeat the stretch with your right leg.

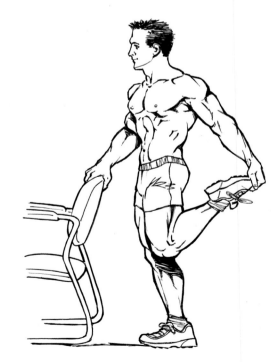

STANDING CALF STRETCH

Find a step or block of wood and place the balls of both feet on the step. Make sure you have something to hold on to in order to help keep your balance. Step up as far as you can go on the balls of your feet, and then slowly lower your heels. Hold that lower position for 15 to 30 seconds, and then rise all the way back up on the balls of your feet. Repeat.

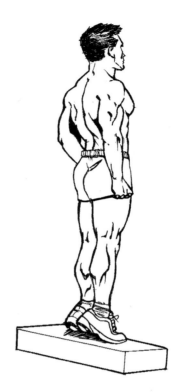

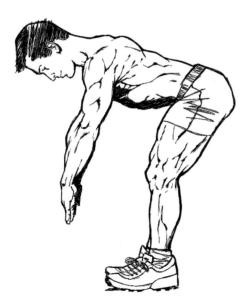

THE TOE TOUCH

Stand with your feet about shoulder-width apart and pointed straight ahead, and keep your back straight. Slowly bend forward from the hips, as if you're trying to touch your toes. Keep your knees slightly bent to avoid stress on the lower back. Let your neck and arms relax to the point where you feel a slight stretch in the lower back, hips, groin and hamstrings. Hold this position for several seconds until you're relaxed. You may even be able to touch your toes.

STRETCHING PRINCIPLES

→ Stretch for 8 to10 minutes overall.

→ Hold each position for 5 to 20 seconds.

→ Be consistent; no long breaks between sessions.

→ No ballistics. Do not bounce.

→ Start a stretch with caution.

→ Stop if you feel pain.

→ Stretch the complete body.

→ Repeat each stretch three times.

→ Invent new stretches for yourself.

→ Don't hold your breath. Breathe in a slow and relaxed manner.

The correct way to stretch is to take your time. Stretching is not a competitive sport. Start with gentleness. Overstretching and stretching with too much enthusiasm can lead to injury. Give yourself time to adjust to the stress and strain. Once you learn how to stretch you will be able to develop your own routine, working more on stubborn areas and less on those already flexible.

Many people who train think stretching is a waste of time. Frequently they push themselves too hard without either warming up or stretching. They end up with an injury. I enjoy my stretching because I love the rewards of feeling flexible. I'm as loose as a goose.

It bears repeating: If you haven't stretched before or haven't done it for a long time, consult your physician before beginning any stretching or exercise program.

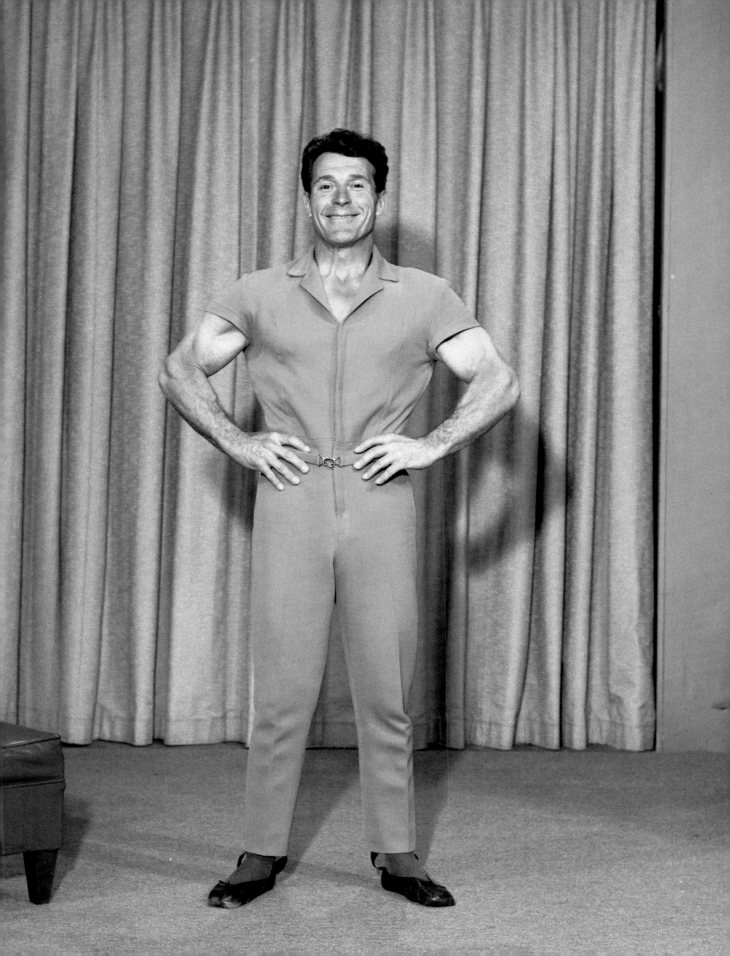

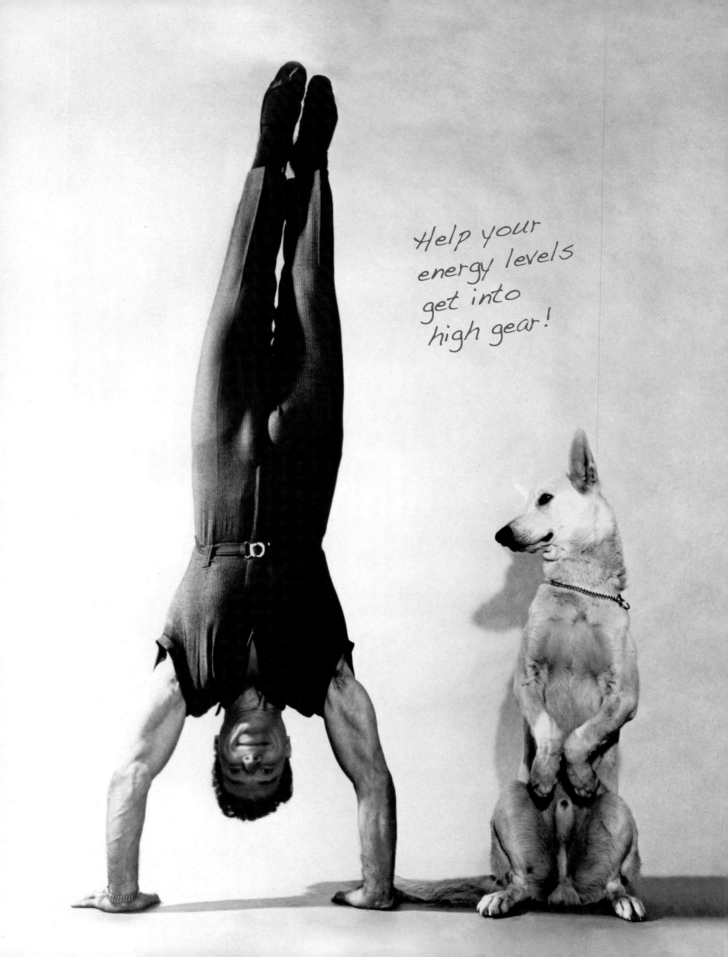

Help your energy levels get into high gear!

CHAPTER ELEVEN

Step 8: Find Some Energy

THE FATIGUE FACTOR

There's probably not a thing clinically wrong with your body, but like millions of other people you nearly always wake up tired. You can't figure it out.

Fatigue is a growing hazard in North America. There's so much to do in a day; it boggles the mind. Didn't our ancestors have to do all the washing by hand, buy groceries daily, sew socks, light fires, make clothes, cut wood, fetch coal, feed the farm animals, collect the eggs, milk the cows, pluck the chickens and skin the rabbits?

Today we have thousands of manufacturers who produce literally millions of so-called time-saving products for our convenience, yet we never have enough time. Where does the day go?

And because the days never seem long enough, there is a tendency to try to add to it by borrowing hours that should be spent in sleep, sleep which when lost can never be regained or made up.

Countless thousands of North Americans visit their doctors every day with western society's most common malady – chronic tiredness. Why does the zest go out of our lives? Do you get overtired well before your bedtime? Do you wake up feeling that you have not completely recharged your batteries?

Everyone gets tired, of course. It's natural and expected. In fact it's desirable. There's a strong satisfaction to feeling pleasantly tired at the end of your day, knowing you are going to retire to your bed for a good night's sleep. Excessive fatigue, however, is debilitating and can result in a sporadic sleep at best. You can wake up in the morning more tired than when you went to bed.

Excessive fatigue is debilitating and can result in a sporadic sleep at best.

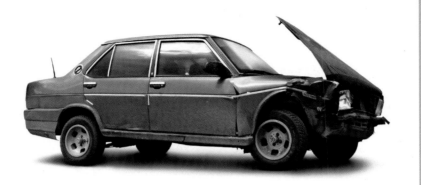

The vast majority of auto accidents are due to fatigue alone or fatigue with alcohol.

You go into sleep deprivation. In time you will become a chronic sufferer, and your body will dig itself deeper and deeper into ill health. First signs will be general listlessness, and then you will find paying attention at office meetings or driving long distances to be "traps" where you can easily nod off. Your resistance to disease will become lowered. The common cold, flu, bronchitis, strep throat, pneumonia and other more serious diseases are likely to strike those suffering from chronic fatigue. The vast majority of auto accidents are due to fatigue alone or fatigue in combination with alcohol. Acts of violence are sometimes committed by those too tired to "know what they were doing."

The principle reason for tiredness is insufficient sleep. However, I am sure you will be shocked to know there are literally hundreds of other causes of tiredness. Little wonder the malady is so common. Even those who get seven to eight hours' sleep can wake up tired because the stresses of the day can lead to restless sleep that just doesn't give the body the deep recuperation it needs.

STEP
8

One of the most common causes of marital disharmony is chronic fatigue.

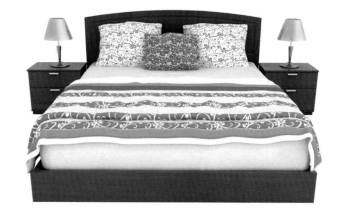

One of the most common causes of marital disharmony, bitterness and bickering is chronic fatigue. Even young couples find their closest moments are frequently forfeited because of tiredness. Typically, while hurriedly readying themselves for a day at the office, married couples will promise each other some loving intimacy come nighttime. But on returning home in traffic, and after housecleaning, supper, driving the kids to sports and watching a TV show or two, the sense of fatigue is so intense that the idea of any sexual activity is, with a sigh of relief, mutually discarded.

The causes of fatigue are legion, ranging from actual lack of sleep to an underactive thyroid to a bad relationship with a fellow colleague at work. In order to meet my responsibility I should say right here that a person who feels perpetually tired should pay a visit to his or her healthcare professional. Chances are you will be given a clean bill of health, but it is nevertheless the correct course to take when one feels "tired all the time." Anemia, poor circulation, blood-pressure abnormalities and more serious illnesses can all cause chronic fatigue. Here are some possible reasons for your fatigue:

EMOTIONS: ANGER AND FEAR

Strong negative emotion is mentally and physically draining, says Dr. Vicky Young, an assistant professor in the department of preventative medicine at the Medical College of Wisconsin. Endeavor to redirect your emotions to your job, or better still to a butt-kicking gym workout.

SAY NO TO TOBACCO

Doctors advise giving up smoking. This wasn't always the case, but doctors think a little more about preventative measures these days. Smoking prevents proper delivery of oxygen to the tissues, and the result is chronic fatigue. Quit today, but don't expect an immediate surge in energy. Nicotine is a stimulant and withdrawal may cause temporary fatigue. My conscience forces me to repeat this: Smoking is one of the very worst things you can do for your health.

KEEP UP WITH YOUR WORKOUTS

Exercise actually builds energy. Hundreds of studies including my own observations after nearly 80 years support this statement, including one by the National Aeronautics and Space Administration. In this study, over 200 employees were placed on regular physical training programs. Ninety percent said they had never felt better. One third said they slept better. But to avoid problems with getting to sleep, try not to exercise later than two hours before bedtime.

STEP

8

Try not to exercise later than two hours before bedtime.

TACKLE ONE THING AT A TIME

Tiredness can come from indecision or lack of planning your day. Dr. David Sheridan MD, an associate professor in the Department of Preventative Medicine at the University of South Carolina School of Medicine says fatigue can come from not taking time each morning to set an agenda for the day. Select goals that are achievable and not overly time consuming. Having to say, "I have so much to do I don't know where to begin," is not a great way to start your inner engine.

> Fatigue can come from not taking time each morning to set an agenda for the day.

EAT A BALANCED BREAKFAST

Breakfast should consist of complex carbohydrates, proteins and fats. However, don't add fat to your menu. They come with the proteins you eat.

Oatmeal or a whole-grain cereal with skim milk makes an excellent start. Add a few berries for good measure. For protein consider a low-fat yogurt, cottage cheese, a small piece of chicken or fish, or an egg-white omelet.

Avoid sugar-loaded cereals that can spike insulin and blood-sugar levels and then drop you down to zero energy.

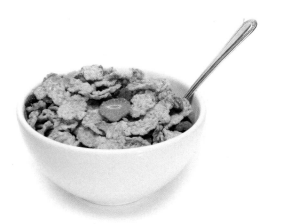

LIMIT YOUR TV TIME

Watching endless hours of TV can lull you into lethargy. Try reading or listening to music. Go for a walk, or do some gardening. Get up off the couch to change things up. Getting super relaxed increases that tired feeling.

ONE A DAY IS OKAY

I've always taken vitamins on a daily basis. Even though I don't miss meals I believe there is a degree of assurance that comes from making sure your vitamin and mineral intake is up to standard. You can't make up for tiredness by eating vitamins, but vitamins in addition to proper food intake can help you feel less tired. For the record, taking vitamins will not offer any defense against heart attack or cancer. But a diet including fruit and veggies can help do just that.

> You can't make up for tiredness by eating vitamins.

TRAVEL CAN BE EXHAUSTING

Air travel, especially through a variety of time zones, can be fatiguing. In some cases excessive tiredness can persist for several days after your plane has landed. Car and bus travel can also increase tiredness, especially when the journey is very long.

TAKING ON EXTRA ACTIVITIES

It's a good idea to delegate, both at work and at home. You can't do everything. Many parents spend time doing dishes, preparing meals, making the beds and sweeping the floor when in fact these jobs can be delegated. Asked to serve on yet another committee? Say no for once. You need time for yourself.

LUNCHTIME BLUES

Going out for a big lunch, especially when a couple of drinks are added to the menu, is no way to beat the tiredness syndrome. Try to keep lunch to a soup and salad and a piece of fruit if possible. Drinks, meat and potatoes, apple pie a la mode and a coffee is one way to guarantee you'll want to sleep at your desk when you get back to the office.

GET 20 WINKS

Personally, I will take a midday nap of 30 minutes if I feel like it.

Naps are not for everybody. Some people just can't get the hang of them. Others feel that there just isn't time. Personally, I will take a midday nap of 30 minutes if I feel like it. Older people who may feel they aren't getting the quality sleep they did in their youth, may benefit from naps. Younger people with hectic work schedules and short nights may benefit from a daily nap. Keep them short and try to nap at the same time each day.

TAKE A VACATION

A trip two or three times a year, even if only for a couple of days, can recharge your batteries. If you can afford it, then getting to sunnier or exotic places during the grayness of winter can be the best medicine in the world. Your energy levels will spring into high gear.

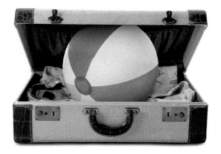

OTHER CAUSES OF
TIREDNESS

→ Sunbathing

→ Depression

→ Room temperature too high

→ Eyestrain

→ Tight clothes

→ Poor lighting conditions

→ Improperly fitting shoes

→ Poor posture

→ Excessive noise

→ Shopping

→ Too much sleep

→ Obesity

→ Pep pills

→ Excessive fresh air

→ Financial worries

→ Loneliness

→ Excessive sexual activity

→ Boredom

→ Overwork at the office

→ Dehydration

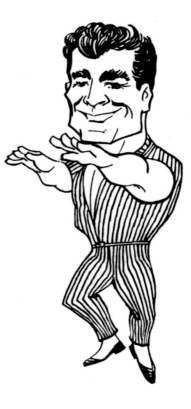

STEP
8

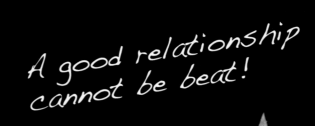

A good relationship
cannot be beat!

CHAPTER TWELVE

Step 9: Be In A Steady Relationship

TWO ARE BETTER THAN ONE

I met my wife Elaine when she was 27. She was a smoker and had a love affair with chocolate doughnuts. She worked for KGO-TV, an ABC-TV station in San Francisco. I joined the station a year after Elaine did, and we actually had to share an office in the newsroom. Elaine was stressed, as are many who work today. She had to run a household, care for two children and hold down a demanding job at the TV station. She told me she was impressed by my huge enthusiasm and unabashed joy at just being alive.

One day in the newsroom she overheard me talking to my director about my lifelong profession of relentlessly pursuing health and fitness. She heard phrases like: "The food you eat today is walking and talking tomorrow," and: "Your waistline is your lifeline." She was becoming intrigued at my energy and enthusiasm for life. One day when she was puffing on a cigarette between taking bites of a chocolate doughnut, I said to her,

"The food
you eat
today is
walking
and talking
tomorrow."

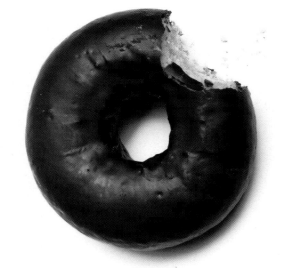

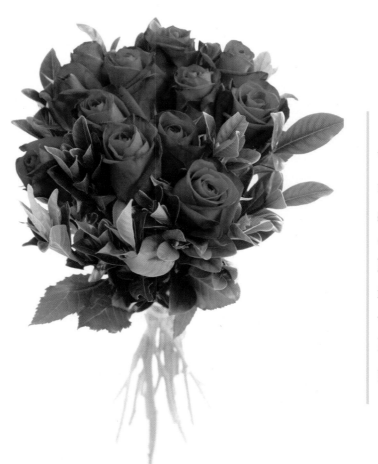

When she
realized I
genuinely
cared about
her she
immediately
wanted to
be a better
person.

"You shouldn't be eating that junk. You should be eating apples, bananas and oranges." She replied, simply, "Oh yeah?" Then I added, "If I didn't like you I wouldn't tell you this." I guess that was the beginning of us as a team, which has lasted to this day.

Elaine once told me that when she realized that I genuinely cared about her she immediately wanted to be a better person – fitter, healthier and more appealing physically. She had gone home that night, stripped off to her birthday suit and stared at her naked body in the mirror. As she put it, she saw her chest sinking into her waistline, and her legs were getting ripples. She felt old and suddenly wanted to be 19 again. Something had to be done.

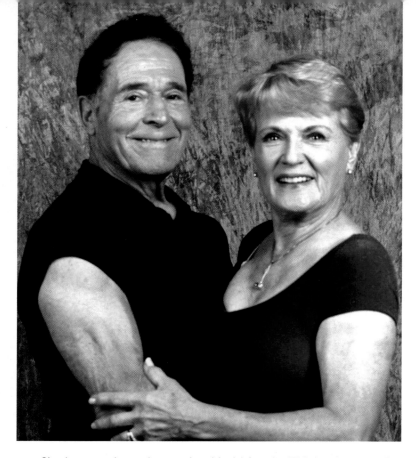

Find the right partner in life, as I did with my wife Elaine.

She began taking classes that I held for the TV employees who showed an interest; she quit smoking and broiled everything she had formerly fried. She cut out all white sugar and white flour and the products manufactured with those ingredients. At my encouragement she took up juicing and felt healthier almost immediately. More on juicing later.

My message is this: A good relationship cannot be beat. Find the right partner in life. Be loyal, and work together as a team. Resist the temptation to let that relationship fall into the trap of resentment, jealousy, envy and bitterness. Be kind to one another. So many married couples let go of that first love and respect that they actually end up hating each other. Don't let things deteriorate. I believe that when two people get together in love and seek a common goal, anything is possible. They can take on the world. Possibilities abound. Nothing is out of reach. My greatest joy has been loving, laughing and working alongside my beautiful Elaine for some 60 wonderful years. I want the same happiness for you.

Remember, our biological drive is several million years older than our intelligence. Don't let your sex drive lead you astray. Right now if you are unattached take great care to choose the right partner. If you have second thoughts over whether or not you could be loyal to your future spouse for the entirety of your marriage, then don't get married. To carry on clandestine affairs turns you into a person who has to constantly lie, fabricate and invent situations, which will inevitably be discovered for what they are. Divorce doesn't just mean losing half your net worth, but should children be in the equation, enormous heartache will be injected into your life. Worst-case scenario? Your kids may come to know and establish some newcomer as their true parent, and you will become the outsider. A stranger to your own children. Life brings its inevitable sorrows without you adding to the milieu because you happen to choose the wrong mate.

On the other side of the coin you can have that blissful, exciting combination of real love, true respect, sexual excitement and a sense of humor that can bring joy to all your married years. As a couple you may take on any project, as Elaine and I did in building a solid following of health-conscious people throughout the world. Our greatest joy and elation comes whenever a formerly out-of-shape follower of our methods greets us in the street, at an airport or restaurant, and tells us how we have changed their lives for the better. Choose your mate wisely and live in a strong, productive and rewarding relationship.

If you have second thoughts over whether you could be loyal to your future spouse, then don't get married.

STEP
9

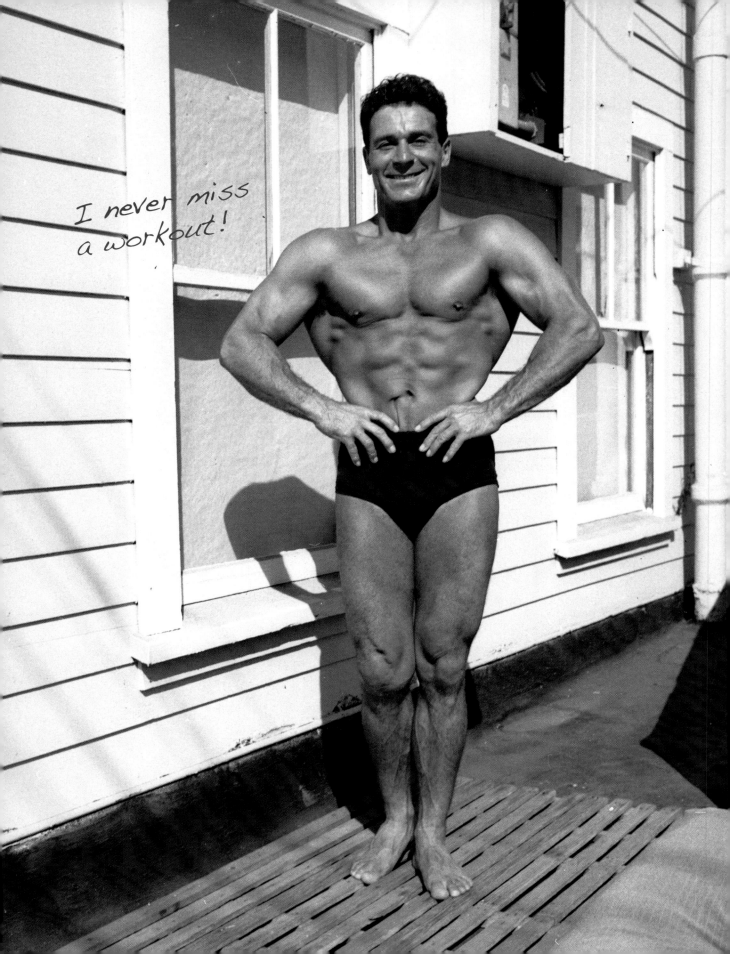

I never miss
a workout!

CHAPTER THIRTEEN

Step 10:
Work Out

MUSCLES ARE BEAUTIFUL – AND USEFUL

I have always trained. I love it. Even now I exercise regularly. I never miss a workout. Today many people spend their spare time watching TV from the soft surrounding of a bed or couch. This is an invitation to lethargy, and when they partner this laziness with the eating of junk food, they're practically inviting a heart attack in middle or later years.

Exercise could almost be called nature's cure-all. It's amazing in its powers. Exercise helps you increase your energy, it cleans out your arteries, improves your posture, increases your mobility, adds muscle and tone, improves strength, builds confidence, burns fat, strengthens bones, hypes your metabolism, augments your flexibility, strengthens your immune system, and shapes your body like nothing else in the world. Hey, you become a more attractive person in every way when you exercise regularly. Even your arteries will thank you.

Exercise is amazing in its powers.

I am a great admirer of the late Winston Churchill. His rousing speeches in time of World War II gave the British people the confidence to stay on course and ultimately prevail against Hitler. But I am most definitely not an advocate of Churchill's oft-quoted line: "When I feel the urge to exercise, I lie down until the feeling goes away." Exercise has been my savior. It has got me to 95 years of age. It has kept me free of disease and made me feel on top of the world ever since I adopted it in my teens. Sometimes you may feel too tired to exercise. We all have moments like that, especially after a long day at the office. Obviously if we are genuinely ill or exhausted then we might have to miss a planned workout, but in most cases one's "tiredness" is little more than a temporary situation – and one that can be immediately changed with a little exercise. Drag yourself to the gym or wherever you exercise and start on something simple. Soon, as your blood starts to circulate, you will be rarin' to go for a full-scale all-out workout.

HOW MUCH WEIGHT?

Whether you decide to work out at home or at a gym you must find the appropriate weight for each exercise. There is no way to know exactly which weight to use without a little trial and error. You never have to go for an all-out gut-bustin' strain. Your repetitions (the number of times you lift a weight) should range between 10 and 20. Your calves or abdominal muscles might respond better to reps in the range of 20 to 30. For most exercises, however, the best number of reps is around 12. This means you should use a weight that challenges you to get 12 reps. However, if you are new to working out, especially if you are on my side of 50, you should probably start with a weight that allows you 20 reps.

Wherever you work out, you must find the appropriate weight for each exercise.

STEP
10

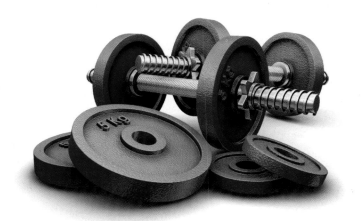

DOCTOR'S OKAY

Get a physician's approval if you are new to exercise, if you are a smoker or if you're over 40. The American College of Sports Medicine recommends that all men and women over 40 about to start an exercise program should visit their health professional and get a stress test that measures both aerobic and muscle condition. Chances are you will get the green light with a congratulatory handshake, but it's always best to be safe. Once you have the okay to work out you will feel on top of the world – ready, willing and able to train for the health, fitness and body shape you desire.

GO EASY TO START

When helping newcomers to training, I insist they not take their exercise efforts to the limit. There has to be a degree of gentleness with your first few workouts. Resist the temptation to suddenly throw yourself into endless furious sessions of strenuous exercise. I want you to coax your muscles into shape, not pound them into a state where they are overtrained. Start slowly. After your first few weeks you will start feeling that you can push yourself harder, and at that time you will likely be ready to do so.

LOSE THE SCALES

Men and women who exercise regularly have no interest in the bathroom scales. If you are not already aware of it, muscle weighs more than fat. This means you can actually weigh more while losing fat because you are adding muscle at the same time your fat is burning off. You are exchanging lighter but bulkier puffy fat for denser, sleek, toned muscle tissue. You are on your way to a healthier, more attractive body. It's the mirror that counts. Throw away the scales.

WEIGHTS ARE GREAT

As men and women get older several things happen, and many of the worse things they experience come from a decrease in muscle tissue. They adopt a tendency to stoop, and women especially may develop osteoporosis. Know this: Weight training will help keep your bones strong. Also, regular weight training guards against injury because resistance strengthens both muscles and tendons. A study published in The Physician and Sports Medicine magazine indicates that female trainers are "somewhat less anxious, neurotic, depressed, angry and confused than the general population."

> **Weight training will help keep your bones strong.**

There's nothing to be afraid of when you take up weight training. There are no undesirable side effects. You won't become muscle bound. You won't look like a Mack truck. Weight training is a healthy pursuit. Men will gain muscle and shape and will lose flab. Women will tone up, develop beautiful form and shed excess fat. Vigorous exercise helps your mind function optimally and conditions you for other sports and activities. Your best life is ready to be lived.

HOW MUCH?

Don't have an hour to work out? That's okay – you do not have to perform an entire routine in one workout, although in earlier days when weight training was in its infancy weight trainers would

> **How often you train and how much you do during each workout is up to you.**

literally train for hours. Now we understand it's okay to split the entire routine into two, three or even four sections throughout the week. How often you train and how much you do during each workout is up to you. You will have to arrange your family commitments, work, school and household chores to fit in with your workouts … or should I say your workouts should be arranged to fit in with your other commitments. The way life is these days you can be sure you will need to juggle some time, but make sure to slot in time for training.

HOW OFTEN?

Training every other day is great, but you can also train two days on, one day off, or any other combination that works for you and results in at least three or four training sessions and at least one rest day per week. Generally speaking, you should exercise each body part from one to three times a week. Training a body part two or three times a week is not better than training once a week, but if you train each body part just once a week you should work those muscles harder, with more sets and possibly more weight. This way of training is not advised until you have been training regularly for a few months.

If you are a complete beginner to weight training I suggest you do only one set of 12 to 15 repetitions for each exercise to start, and work each body part two or three times a week. As you progress, you can add sets, increase weights, and reduce repetitions if you would like to progress.

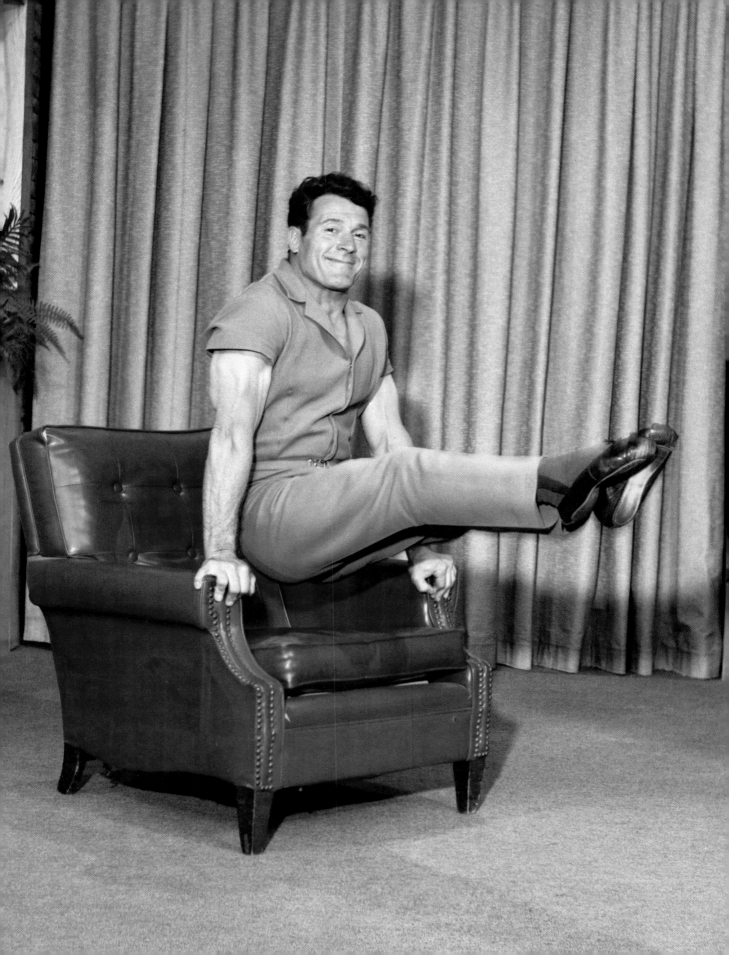

YOUR HOME TRAINING ROUTINE

The following is a functional weight-training routine that can be performed by men or women at home. All you need is a flat exercise bench and some dumbbells. Most sporting goods stores sell dumbbells, and they are not expensive. Considering that they last for a lifetime, they are an economical investment.

THIGHS

Wide-leg squats

Lunges

CALVES

Dumbbell calf raises

SHOULDERS

Upright rows

Bent-over flyes

CHEST

Lying dumbbell presses

Dumbbell flyes

BACK

Dumbbell bent-over rows

Single-arm dumbbell rows

ABDOMINALS

Toes-to-ceiling raises

Bent-knee tucks

TRICEPS

Triceps kickbacks

Seated dumbbell extensions

BICEPS

Standing hammer curls

Seated alternating curls

THIGHS
WIDE-LEG SQUATS

Stand, holding one dumbbell with both hands at about pelvis level, feet about a yard apart and toes pointing outward at 10 to 2. Keeping back straight, squat down until your thighs are parallel to the floor. Stand up, keeping your back straight. If you are a complete beginner, use a light weight and complete one set of 15 reps. If you are used to exercise, use a heavier weight and do 3 sets of 8 to 12 reps.

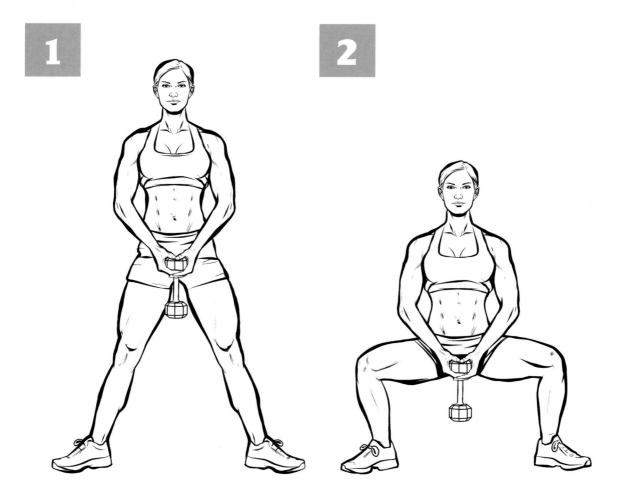

THIGHS
LUNGES

Stand, feet together, back straight. Hold dumbbells at arms' length in a relaxed manner. Step quite far forward with your right foot, allowing your body to drop as you do so.

Bring the knee of your rear leg down close to the floor. Make sure the knee of your front leg does not extend past your toe. Push off with your front leg and return to the starting position. Repeat, with left leg coming forward. To help prevent a rounded back, look at a spot on the wall opposite throughout the entire exercise. Do a single set of 15 to 20 reps per leg if you are a beginner. An advanced trainer can do up to five or six sets.

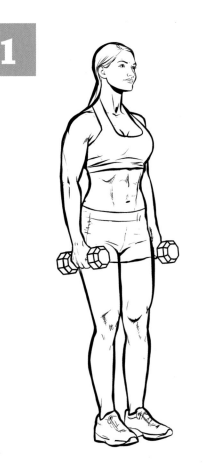

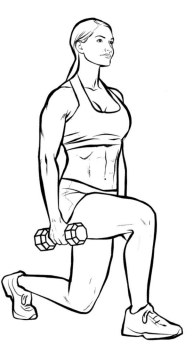

CALVES
DUMBBELL CALF RAISES

Stand on a sturdy block or bench, holding a dumbbell relaxed at arm's length in each hand. Rise up on your toes as far as you can go, and then lower your heels down further than the block or bench you are standing on. Feel a good stretch through your calves. Rise up again on your toes. Beginners should do one set of 20 to 25 reps. Advanced trainers can start with a set such as this to warm up, and then pick up a heavier weight and do three sets or more of 15 reps to 20 reps.

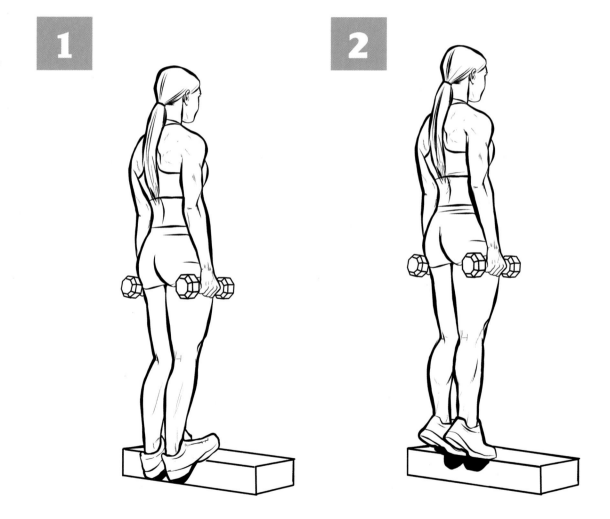

SHOULDERS
UPRIGHT ROWS

Hold two dumbbells at arms' length at the front of your body. Standing straight and moving only your arms, lift the dumbbells simultaneously until they reach upper-chest level. Repeat for a total of 15 reps if you are a beginner, and do 3 sets of 15 reps if you are advanced.

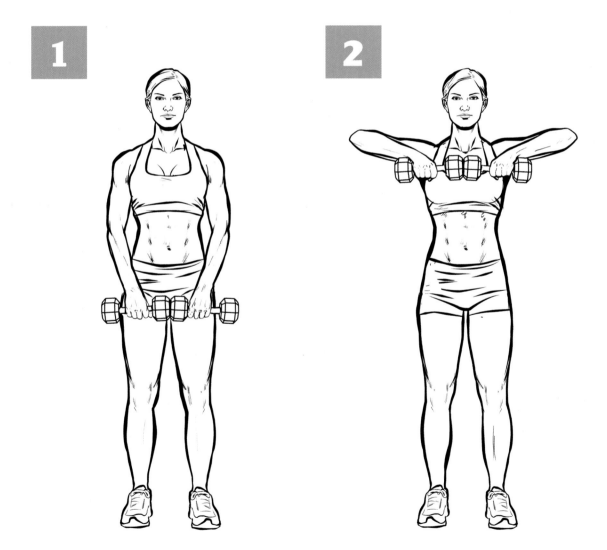

SHOULDERS
BENT-OVER FLYES

This exercise hits your rear shoulders – an area often neglected. Sit at the edge of a bench or chair. Leaning far forward, pick your dumbbells up off the floor and, still bent over, lift the weights directly out to your sides until arms are level with your body. Keep your arms bent slightly throughout. Feel the muscles at the rear of your shoulders doing the work. Use a light weight, especially to start off. Beginners can do a set of 12 to 15 reps. If you are an advanced trainer, do 3 sets of 10 to 12 reps.

1　　　　　　　　　　**2**

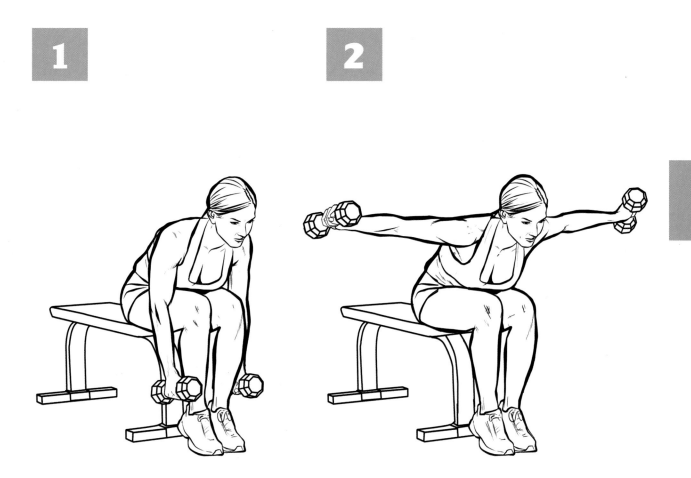

CHEST
LYING DUMBBELL PRESSES

Lie back on a bench, feet on the floor for support, holding two dumbbells above your chest, arms straight. Bring the weights down to your sides, keeping them level. You should feel a stretch in your chest. Your forearms should remain perpendicular to the floor throughout the exercise. If you are a beginner you can do sets of 10 to 15 reps, and then as you progress, work your way up in weight and sets and down in reps, to 3 or 4 sets of 6 to 10 reps.

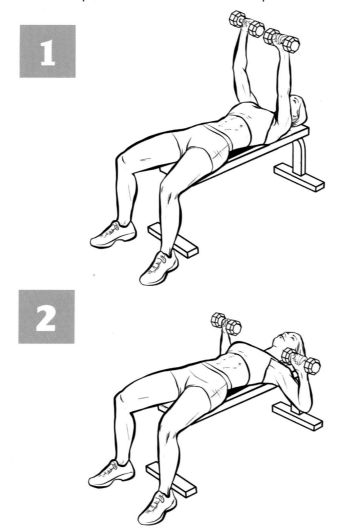

CHEST
DUMBBELL FLYES

Lie on a bench on your back, feet on the floor, holding two dumbbells. Bring your arms out to the sides, elbows slightly bent, until you feel a stretch through your chest. Keeping arms slightly bent, bring dumbbells together above your chest. The movement is often described as "hugging a tree." Bring the dumbbells back to the starting position at your sides, and repeat. Do one set of 10 to 15 reps as a beginner, and 3 sets of 6 to 10 reps if advanced.

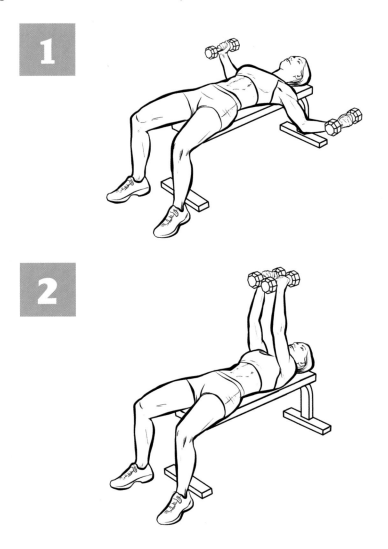

BACK
DUMBBELL BENT-OVER ROWS

Stand, feet shoulder-width apart, holding two dumbbells. Bending your knees slightly, bend over until your body is close to parallel with the floor. Do NOT round your back! If you do, you risk injury. The trick to keeping your back safely arched is to keep your butt up in the air and your eyes focused across the room. It might feel silly, but it works! Now, keeping your body still, lift the dumbbells to your sides simultaneously, keeping them level. Bring them up as far as possible without twisting your body. Feel the squeeze in your back. Lower and repeat. As a beginner, do a set of 12 to 15 and work your way up to 3 sets of 8 to 12 as you progress.

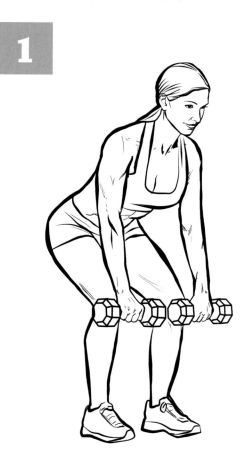

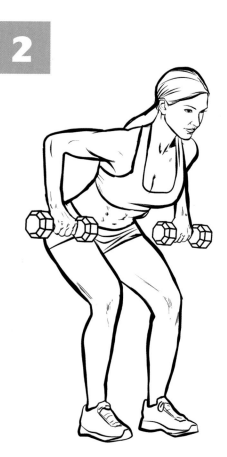

BACK
SINGLE-ARM DUMBBELL ROWS

Stand holding a dumbbell in one hand, and step forward with the foot opposite to the hand in which you are holding a dumbbell. Lean over and place your other hand on the thigh of the forward leg, supporting your body weight. Keep your back arched rather than rounded. Hold your stomach in. Stretch the arm with the weight down as far as you can while keeping your body in position. You should feel a nice stretch in your lat (the muscle at the side of your back). Lift the weight high up to your side, feeling the back muscles working. Beginners do one set of 10 to 15 for each side, advanced do 3 sets of 8 to 12.

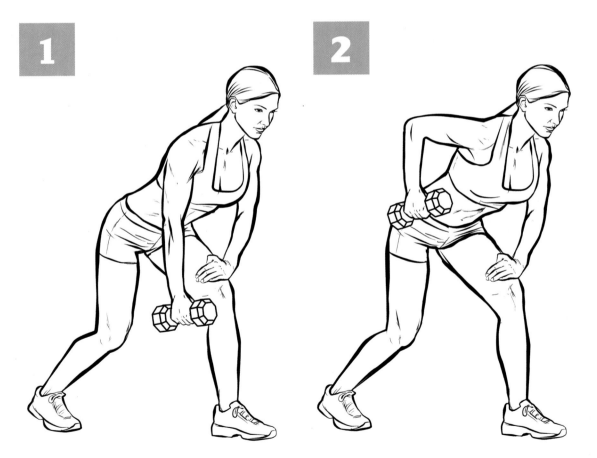

ABDOMINALS
TOES-TO-CEILING RAISES

Lie on a flat bench. Grasp the sides of the bench beside your head to aid in stability. Keeping your back flat, raise your legs straight up, so your toes are pointed toward the ceiling. Leading with your heels and using your abdominal muscles, raise your lower body straight up. Your legs should not swing forward, but should remain vertical throughout the movement. Lower your hips to the bench, keeping your legs in the same vertical position. Repeat as many times as you can. Work your way up to 25-rep sets.

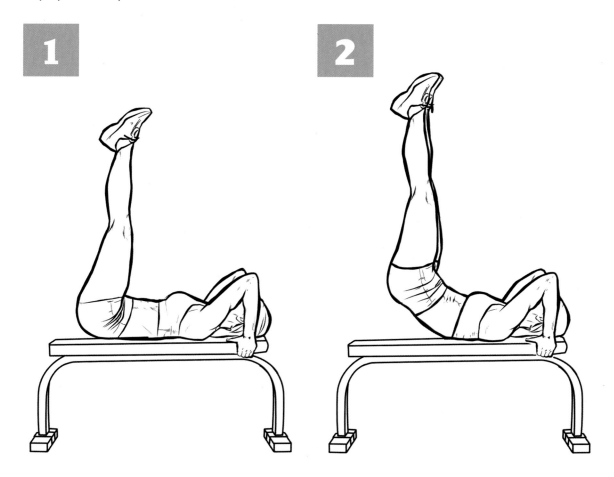

ABDOMINALS
BENT-KNEE TUCKS

Sit sideways on a bench, grasping the side. Lean back and straighten your legs, using your hands to help stay balanced. Keeping your abs tight and back straight, bring your knees in toward your chest and then push them out again so your legs are straight. Do not touch the floor with your feet between reps, but rather keep the tension in your abdominal area. Complete as many reps as you can. Work your way up to 25-rep sets.

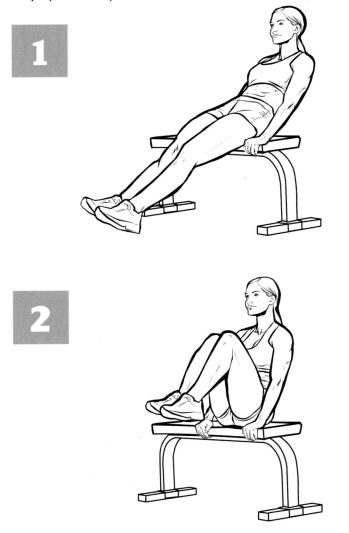

TRICEPS
TRICEP KICKBACKS

Standing, step forward with one foot. Bend over to nearly parallel to the floor, making sure to keep your back flat or arched and not rounded. Hold a dumbbell at the side of your rear leg, and lean on the forward leg with your other hand for support. Bending your arm, bring the weight up so your forearm is perpendicular to the floor. Keeping your upper arm still and close to your body, swing your lower arm back with control, straightening your arm completely. Again with control, bring your lower arm back to starting position. Beginners should aim for one set of 10 to 15 reps. Work up to 3 sets of 10 to 15 as you progress. This is not a big-weight exercise.

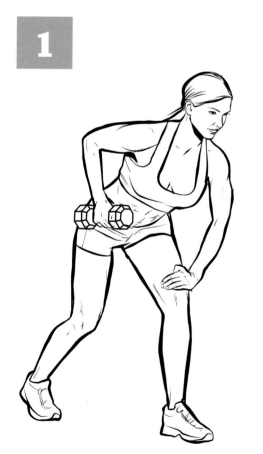

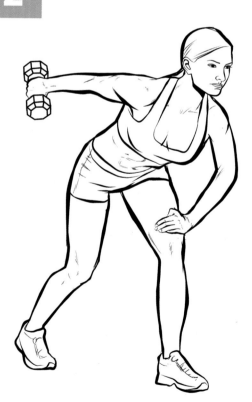

TRICEPS
SEATED DUMBBELL EXTENSIONS

Sit sideways on a flat bench, holding a dumbbell in one hand. Lift the dumbbell and lower behind your head. Your upper arm should be perpendicular to the floor and close in to your head throughout this exercise. Once the dumbbell is in position behind your head, straighten your arm completely, and then lower again with control. Remember to keep your upper arm still. If you cannot keep your upper arm directly beside your head throughout this movement, you can try using a lighter weight or you can hold your upper arm with your free hand. Again, beginners can do one set of 10 to 15 reps and advanced trainers can do 3 sets of 10 to 15 reps.

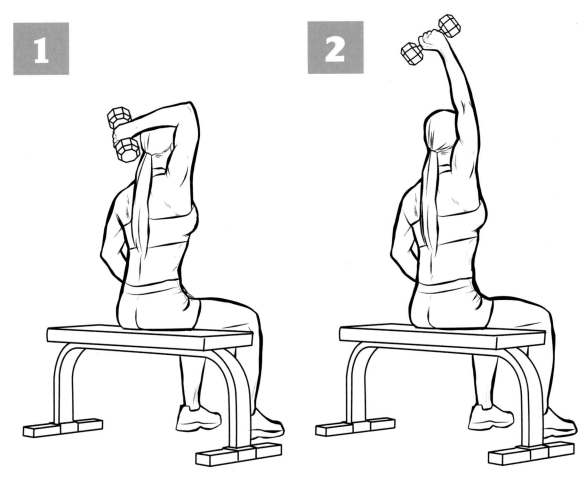

BICEPS
STANDING HAMMER CURLS

Stand, feet shoulder-width apart, dumbbells held at arms' length at your sides. Keeping the palms of your hands facing each other and your upper arms tight to your body throughout this exercise, lift the dumbbells by bending your elbows. Bring the weights up to shoulder level, and then down again with control. Do not snap or swing the weights up and down, as this can damage your tendons. Repeat until you have completed one set of 15 as a beginner, or 3 sets of 8 to 12 as an advanced trainer.

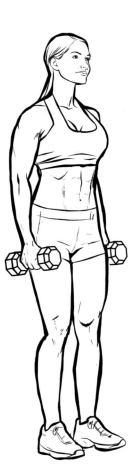

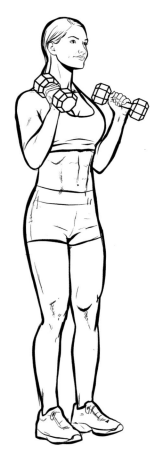

BICEPS
SEATED ALTERNATING CURLS

Sit at the end of your bench, dumbbells held relaxed at arms' length at your sides. Lift one dumbbell by bending your elbow, keeping your upper arm still and close to your body. Turn your arm as you lift, so at the top of the movement your palm faces your body. Once you reach your shoulder with the dumbbell, begin to lower that dumbbell with control as you begin to lift the other dumbbell. When one dumbbell is down, the other is up. This should be a rhythmic movement and not a swinging movement. Keep your body and upper arms still throughout. Do one set of 15 as a beginner or 3 sets of 8 to 12 if you are an advanced trainer.

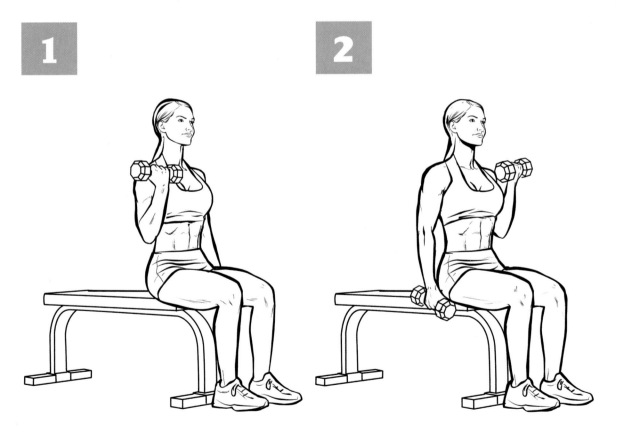

YOUR GYM TRAINING ROUTINE

Men and women vary a great deal here. Women train with much more care and concern about performing an exercise correctly with good form. Men, on the other hand, usually throw good form to the wind and try to lift as much as possible, twisting, swinging and contorting the body to get the weight up. This can lead to injury. A severe muscle tear can take months to heal properly. Weights should be lifted at moderate speed, not super slow or excessively fast.

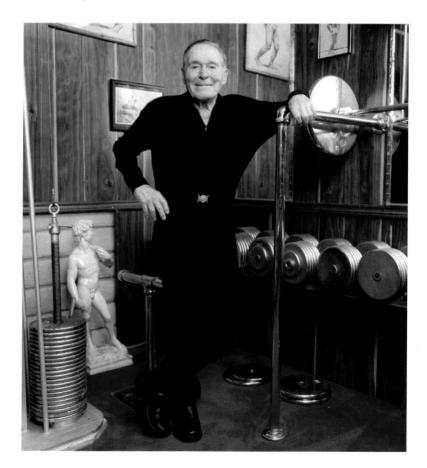

The following is your gym training routine. The same recommendations of sets, reps, intensity and frequency apply.

THIGHS

Smith-machine squats

Leg curls

CALVES

Standing calf-machine heel raises

Seated calf-machine heel raises

GLUTES

Low-pulley bench kickbacks

SHOULDERS

Seated dumbbell shoulder presses

Lateral raises

Bent-over flyes

BACK

Lat-machine pulldowns

Low pulley rows

ABDOMINALS

Captains-chair knee raises

Reverse crunches

CHEST

Incline dumbbell presses
   (35° angle to the bench)

Cable crossovers

BICEPS

Incline dumbbell curls

Preacher bench barbell curls

TRICEPS

Lying triceps barbell extensions

Triceps pushdowns

STEP
10

THIGHS
SMITH-MACHINE SQUATS

Set the bar of the Smith machine at a level just lower than your shoulders. Load an appropriate weight on the bar. Step underneath the bar until it rests on your traps (the meaty part of your shoulder area). Stand up, turn the bar until it becomes unlatched, and then bend your knees to squat down until your upper legs are about parallel to the floor. Stand up again but do not latch the bar. Keep up this smooth up-and-down motion until the end of your set, at which time you will lift the bar slightly higher and turn it until it latches again.

This machine is easy for anyone to use, safe, and allows positions that would be impossible with a regular barbell squat. It's a good idea to get someone at the gym to show you how to use it if you've never done so. Whether you are a man or a woman, you can do anything from very light to very heavy squats. However, make sure to work your way up to heavy weights, and anyone doing heavier weights should do one or two warm-up sets first. One set of 12 to 20 is fine for beginners.

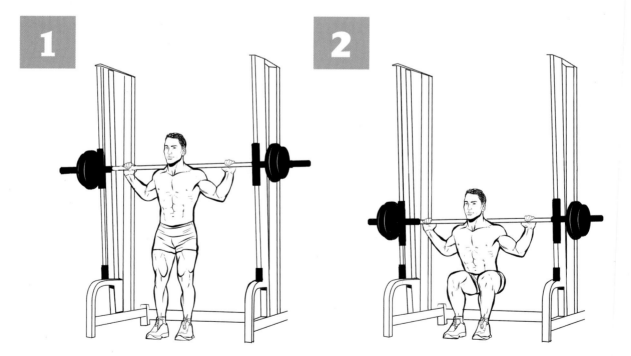

THIGHS
LEG CURLS

Your gym might have a standing machine, as shown, but it's more likely to have a lying machine. If you have a standing machine, then stand straight on the right platform, holding the machine for balance. Select the weight you would like. Place your left ankle to the front of the roller. Bend your left leg until the roller reaches the top position, and lower with control. Do a set for one leg, then stand on the other platform and repeat the instructions for the other leg. Do 1 to 3 sets of 12 to 15 reps per leg.

If you have a lying leg curl machine, then lie face down, slide your feet under the rollers and grasp the handles. Bend your legs, bringing the rollers toward your buttocks. Most machines these days are angled to allow for a natural curve of the body at the hips. A flat bench may cause lower-back strain when performing this exercise. Do 1 to 3 sets of 12 to 15 reps.

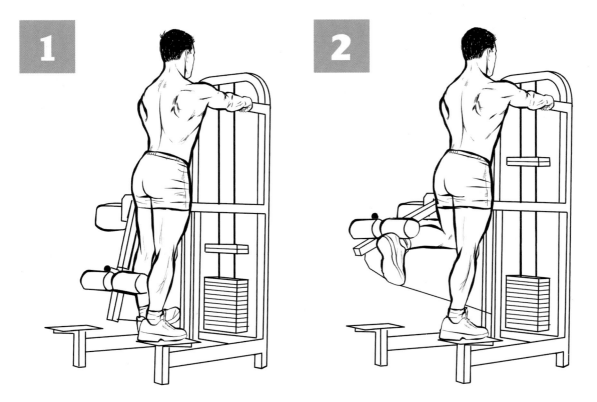

CALVES
STANDING CALF-MACHINE HEEL RAISES

Select the weight you would like. Stand on the machine's platform. You will have to bend slightly to get underneath the shoulder pads. Once you have set your shoulders securely under the pads, stand straight. Go up as far as you can on your toes, then lower, stretching your calves as far as they will go. Keep up this up-and-down motion for at least 15 reps and up to 25. Calves take a lot of weight and a lot of work. Do one set as a beginner, and 3 sets as an advanced trainer.

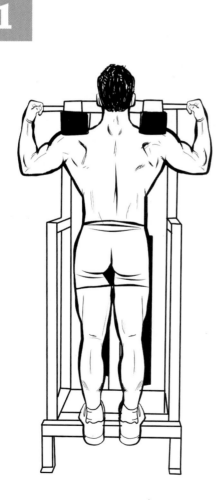

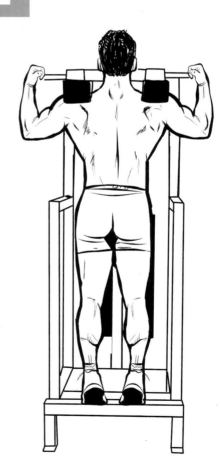

CALVES
SEATED CALF-MACHINE HEEL RAISES

This machine develops a different calf muscle – the soleus, which lies beneath the diamond-shaped gastrocnemius, which is what we usually think of as the calf.

Load the machine with the appropriate weights. Sit on the chair and slide your knees under the pad. Lift the pad by going up on your toes. Release the catch. Lower your heels down below the footrests. Continue with this up-and-down motion, making sure to go as high and low as possible to get the full range of movement. Aim for about 15 reps. Do one set as a beginner, or 3 sets if you are advanced.

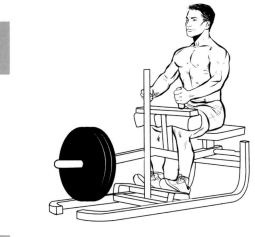

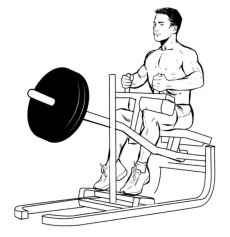

GLUTES
LOW-PULLEY BENCH KICKBACKS

This is one of the best exercises out there for creating a nice, round butt. Kneel with one leg on a flat bench next to a pulley machine. Strap the cuff handle around the other ankle. Make sure the bench is far enough from the cable that you feel resistance even when your leg is in the forward position. Rise up so you can swing your straight leg back without hitting the floor. Allow your leg to gently pull to its most forward position, and then forcefully swing it back until parallel to the floor. Bring your leg back to the forward position with control – don't let it snap back. Do a set of 10 to 15 reps, then switch to the other leg. Do 3 sets if you are an advanced trainer.

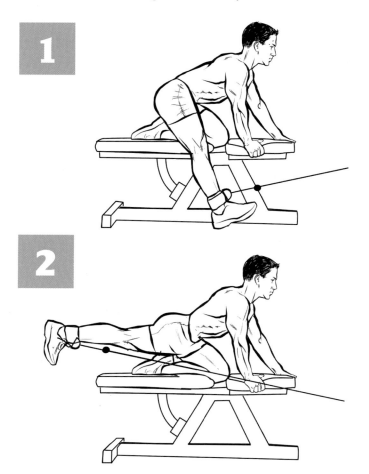

SHOULDERS
SEATED DUMBBELL SHOULDER PRESSES

Sit at the end of a bench, dumbbells either on the floor, if heavy, or in your hands in a relaxed position. Being careful not to round your back, hoist the dumbbells up to shoulder level, and then push up until your elbows almost lock out. Lower to shoulder level and repeat. At the end of your set, place dumbbells on the floor while you rest. One set of 12 to 15 reps is enough for beginners, 3 sets of 8 to 15 for advanced trainers.

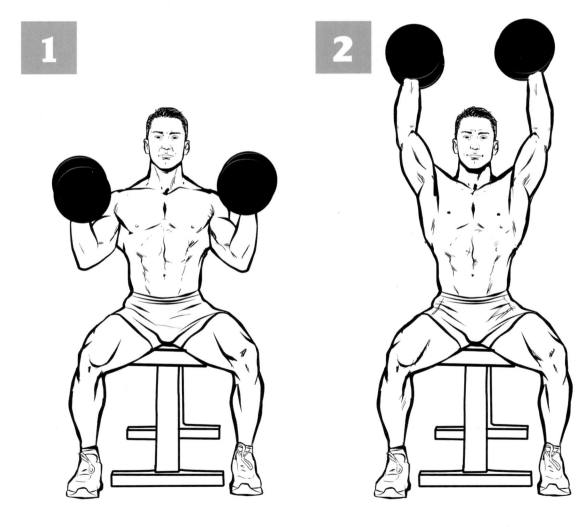

SHOULDERS
LATERAL RAISES

Stand, feet shoulder-width apart, dumbbells held to the front. Keeping your elbows slightly bent, simultaneously raise both arms from the shoulders until your arms are slightly above shoulder level. Bring back down with control. Do not swing your body to get the weights up – feel your shoulder muscles (deltoids) doing the work. If you cannot complete this move with just shoulder-muscle power, decrease the weight. Do 10 to 15 reps, one set for beginners, 3 sets for advanced.

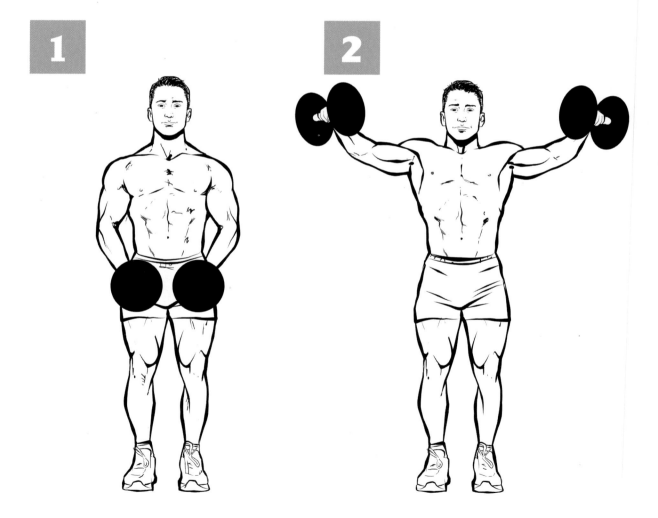

SHOULDERS
BENT-OVER FLYES

Stand, feet shoulder-width apart, dumbbells in hand. Bend forward until your upper back is near parallel to the floor. Make sure your back is arched or straight and not rounded. To do this, stick your butt in the air, pull your stomach in and look ahead. Hold dumbbells nearly at arms' length, but with a very slight bend in the elbows. Simultaneously raise both arms straight out from the shoulders until your arms are level with your body. Feel the muscles of your rear shoulder doing the work. Keep your body stable and move only your arms. Bring back down with control. Do 10 to 15 reps, one set for beginners, 3 sets for advanced.

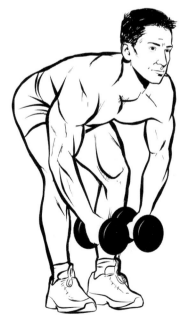

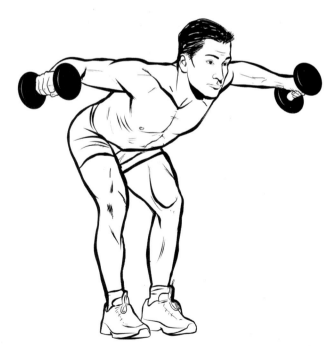

BACK
LAT-MACHINE PULLDOWNS

Sit on the chair of the lat machine, knees secured under the pad. Set the pin to the appropriate weight. Reach up and grasp the handle with a wide grip. (You may have to come up out of your seat in order to accomplish this.) Sit up fairly straight, and bring the bar down to shoulder level just in front. Squeeze. Allow bar back up, with control, to almost the top. Do not come out of your seat, but rather use the force to stretch your lat muscles. One set of 12 to 15 reps for beginners, 3 sets of 8 to 12 for advanced.

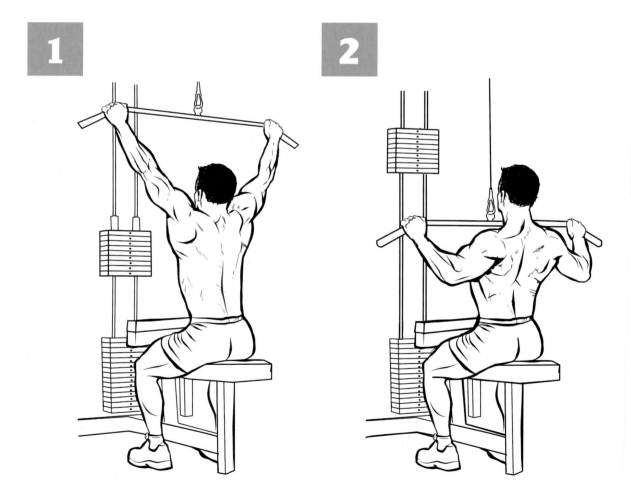

BACK
LOW PULLEY ROWS

Sit on the chair of the low-pulley cable area and adjust the pin to the appropriate weight. Rest your feet on the footrest, lean forward, grasp the handle and sit back, being careful of your lower back while doing so. Keeping your back arched and not rounded, pull the handle in to your lower chest area. Squeeze your back muscles, and then allow the weight back as you bend forward. Do not put the weight right back down — keep some resistance on the cable. Repeat the movement. Beginners can do a set of about 12 to 15 reps, advanced trainers can do 3 sets of 8 to 12.

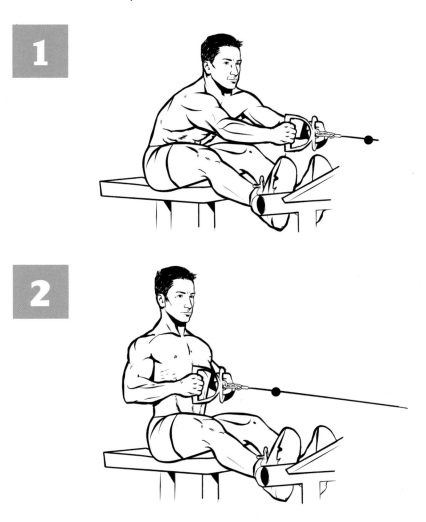

ABDOMINALS
CAPTAINS-CHAIR KNEE RAISES

Climb onto the captain's chair apparatus, facing out. Stand on the footrests and place your fore-arms on the padded armrests, grabbing the support handles. Press your back against the backrest. Once you are settled in position, lift your legs up, bending your knees as you do so, using only your abdominal muscles. Your buttocks should come off the backrest at the top of the exercise. Lower your legs, keeping the abdominals working all the way. Do not place your feet on the rests; instead complete another rep. Do as many as you can, working your way up to 25 reps. Once you can do 25, start doing 2 sets.

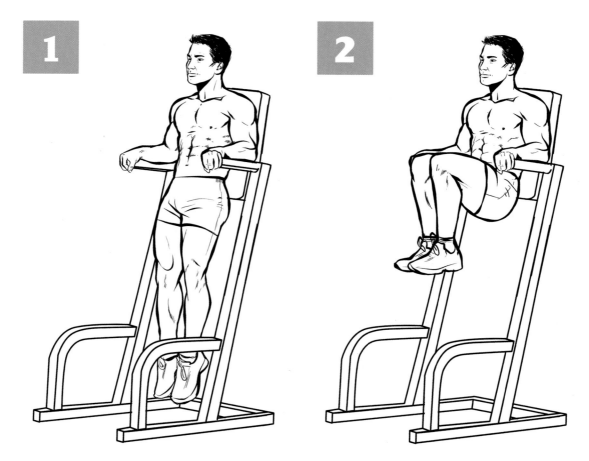

ABDOMINALS
REVERSE CRUNCHES

Lie on a flat bench, buttocks just over the edge and feet on the floor. Grasp the sides of the bench by your head for stability. Keeping knees bent, bring your legs toward your upper body, and then slowly back down, letting your toes just kiss the floor. Do not swing – make sure your abs are doing the work and not momentum. If you do this exercise correctly it works wonders – especially for the hard-to-reach lower abs. Do 10 to 25 reps.

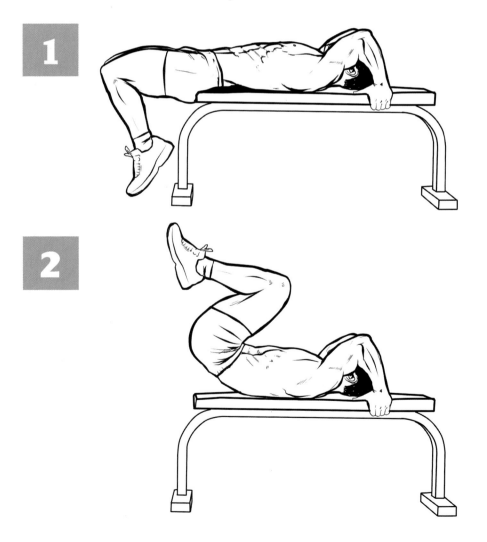

CHEST
INCLINE DUMBBELL PRESSES (35° ANGLE TO BENCH)

Set an adjustable bench so the back is angled at 35 degrees. Rest your dumbbells on the floor and sit on the bench's chair. Lean forward, grab the dumbbells and lie back on the bench, bringing the dumbbells to your shoulder level. Do this all in one fluid motion. Press the dumbbells straight up toward the ceiling, and bring in together so the dumbbells form a straight line. Bring back to shoulder level, making sure to feel a stretch in your chest. Do a set of 12 to 15 if you are a beginner, and 3 sets of 8 to 12 if you are a more advanced trainer.

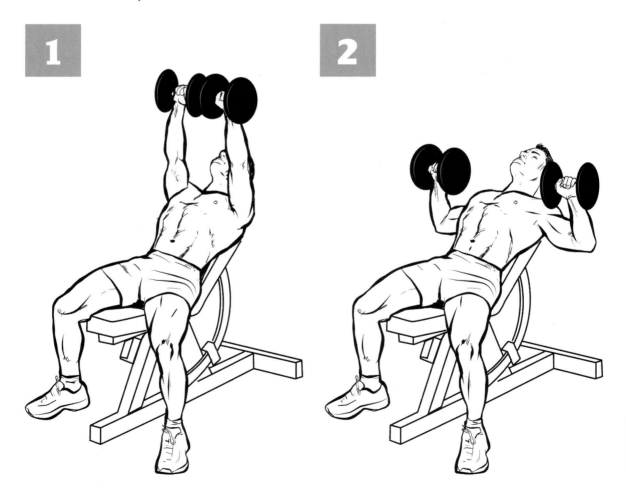

CHEST
CABLE CROSSOVERS

For this exercise your gym will need to have a cable crossover apparatus. Make sure the handles are level and the two weight-stack pins are set at the same weight. Grab hold of one handle and step across to the grab the other handle, as you will not be able to reach them both at the same time. Step into the very middle of the apparatus, set yourself in a solid stance, feet shoulder-width apart, knees slightly bent and upper body leaning slightly forward. Allow your arms to drift back into a position that stretches your chest, but keep your elbows bent. Push the handles together in a "hugging a tree" motion. You could also do as the name suggests and cross your hands in front of each other. Allow your hands to drift back again, keeping arms stiff and slightly bent, and repeat. You can do about 15 reps of this exercise – one set for beginners and 3 for advanced trainers.

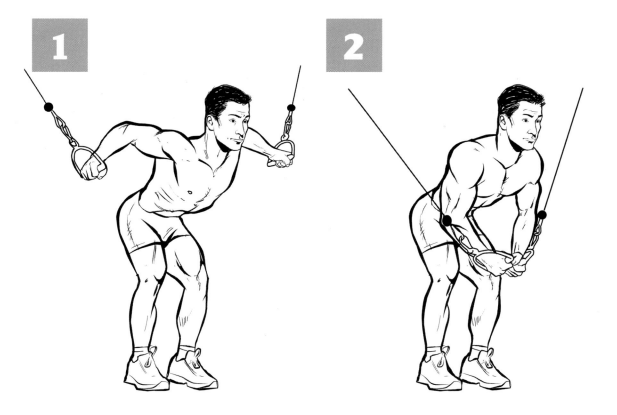

BICEPS
INCLINE DUMBBELL CURLS

Set an incline bench to anywhere from a 45- to 60-degree angle. Sit on the chair of the bench, grab hold of your dumbbells and lean back, allowing your hands to drop to the sides. Turn your hands so the palms face forward, and curl the weights up by bending your elbows, bringing the weights up to about shoulder level. Lower them with control. Do a set of 15 reps if you are a beginner, and 3 sets of 6 to 12 if you are advanced.

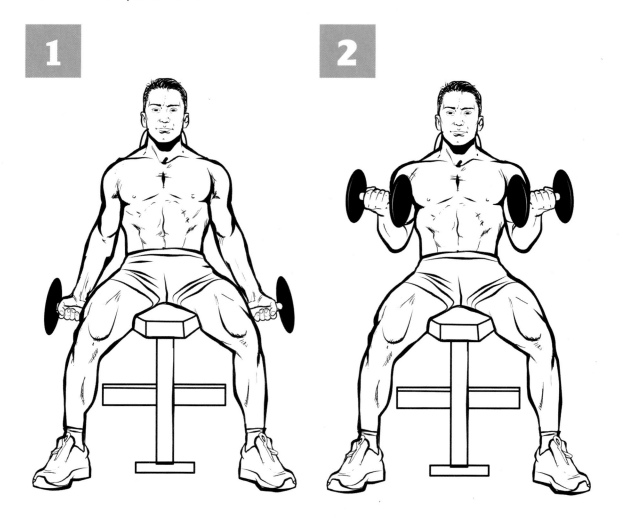

BICEPS
PREACHER BENCH BARBELL CURLS

Place a barbell on the rack of the preacher bench. It's normally best to use an EZ-curl bar, as depicted in the illustration. EZ-curl bars allow your wrists to move in a more natural line when performing this exercise. Place the desired weights on the barbell and climb around to the other side of the bench. Stand tight against the pad, with the top of the pad close to your underarms. Reach forward, grab hold of the bar and curl up. You will need to use less weight than you would standing and curling a barbell, because your biceps muscles are well isolated. Do one to 3 sets of 8 to 15 reps.

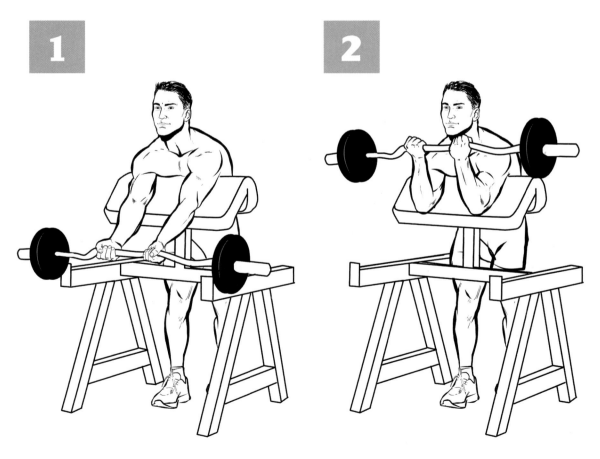

TRICEPS
LYING TRICEPS BARBELL EXTENSIONS

This exercise is one of the best for improving your triceps, the big muscle at the back of your upper arm. Load a barbell with an appropriate weight. Lie on a flat bench, looking up, feet on the floor, and bring your barbell into position: your arms straight and locked out above your shoulders. Bending your elbows but keeping your upper arms as still as possible, lower the weight to your forehead and then push back up, straightening your arms. You should use a spotter (someone to help) with this exercise, especially in the beginning. While you can work your way up to big weights in this exercise, use lighter weights until you get a good idea of the weight you can handle – they don't call this the skullcrusher for nothing! Start with one set of 12 to 15 reps and work your way up to 3 sets of 8 to 12 reps.

1 **2**

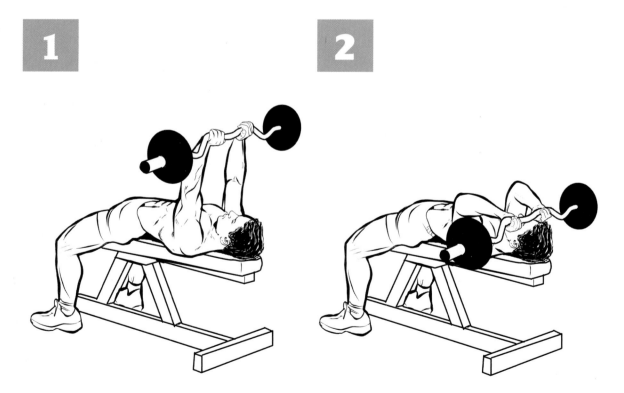

TRICEPS
TRICEPS PUSHDOWNS

Stand at a cable apparatus, pulley in the top position. Set the pin in the desired setting and put a V-handle on the carabiner. Reach up, pull the handle to position at lower chest level, and set your body – feet shoulder-width apart, upper arms tight to your torso. Moving your lower arms only, press the V-handle down until your arms are straight. Squeeze the muscle and then slowly allow back up to chest level. Do a set of 12 to 15 reps to start, then work your way up to 3 sets of 8 to 12 reps.

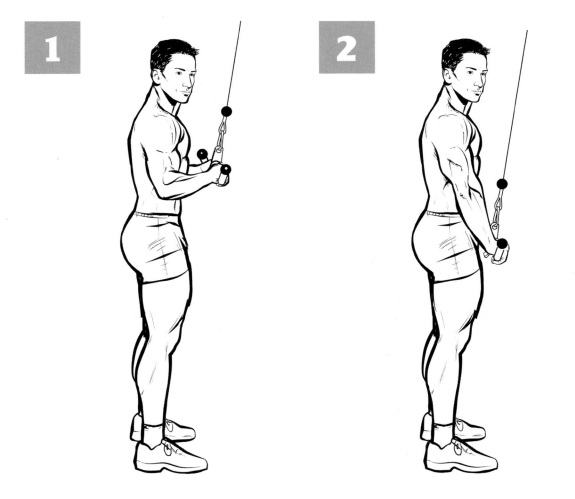

Be positive and confident about making changes!

CHAPTER FOURTEEN

Step 11:
Never Retire

When you slow down too much, you come to a stop.

I guess when you work at something you love it isn't work. I'm lucky that way. I've been involved with fitness just about all my life and I've loved every minute. It's been a blast — and continues to be a blast.

I work out regularly and I follow a diet of natural wholesome foods, both of which habits I recommend to one and all. I have no interest in retiring whatsoever. I will push on till my last breath. Because I have lived so long I have known literally hundreds of individuals who have retired. Some in their late 40s or early 50s. Unless you find another interest, retirement is getting up and going to bed, with eating and television in between. Statistics indicate that most men who retire die within five years of retiring. Not good odds, is it? A good retirement to me is about two weeks.

Okay, so you are in your 50s and you've spent 25 years hacking away two miles underground in a coalmine. Take your retirement. That and other employment of similar ilk are worth retiring

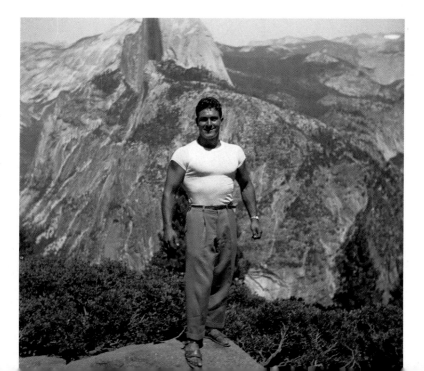

> **Statistics indicate that most men who retire die within five years of retiring.**

from. But even so, I suggest you get another less physical job, or at the very least a demanding and challenging hobby. We must all have an active interest in life. Stagnating on the couch watching game shows on TV is not the way to go. Besides, this type of lazy retirement ruins that jubilant Friday afternoon feeling. The exultation of the weekend is never to be felt again.

The only people who really enjoy their retirement are those who have an all-encompassing interest that substitutes totally for their time spent in the workforce. Even so there's a big difference. As a retiree, unlike when you were working at the office, it isn't mandatory for anyone to listen to you any more. That alone can lessen your sense of importance. You may even feel that you have no purpose in the machinations of society.

I have known scores of people who have been utterly excited over the prospect of retiring. "Now I can travel." "Now I'll have time with my family." "Now I can clean my teeth after every meal." But what happens after a few months? They start missing being at work. I have known gym owners who have rushed to reopen within a couple of years of retiring. One 64-year-old publisher, after selling his fitness magazine, couldn't bear staying at home with nothing to do. A year later he was back into publishing. Why? "I miss it!" he told me. "But you were always grumbling about the price of paper, the problems with staff and freelance writers," I said. "I know, I know," he replied. "But I missed all that too."

The only profession I know where people don't retire is acting. It's true that actors don't retire; they just get offered fewer roles. Gee, I must have been taking some funny pills this morning. I crack me up!

> **As a retiree you may feel that you have no purpose in the machinations of society.**

One solution to dodging full retirement is to retire partially. Some people find that taking a two- or three-day-a-week job suits them just fine. They feel useful, get out of the house, earn some cash, and yet still have time for enjoying freedom they can't experience when locked into a full-time vocation.

How is your current job? Are you stressed at the abundance of work? Frustrated with fellow staff members? Is your commute too stressful and time consuming? Remember we only have one life, and believe me it's a happy day when you actually enjoy your work. Right now at 95 years of age I have a full schedule of seminars, book signings, answering e-mails, swimming and exercising, along with promoting my juicer and the belief in juicing. In addition to that I am in the middle of writing this book. How many 95-year-olds write a book? How do I do it? Answer: I do it when I want to. Usually that translates to my writing about a thousand words a day – sometimes more, sometimes less. And if I feel like missing a couple of days, so be it. I don't lose any sleep over it, but then I don't go for long periods without writing, either. That would take me right out of the creative loop. Writing for me is fun. It's the opposite of working out, or pulling 70 boats across the San Francisco Bay on my 70th birthday. Writing is a release. Besides, I enjoy knowing that my writing can influence people and get them active and healthy. What better reward is there than to know that what you are doing is helping people live longer, and enjoy their lives to the fullest. It's mind blowing.

> *I've been involved with fitness just about all my life and I've loved every minute of it. It's a blast!*

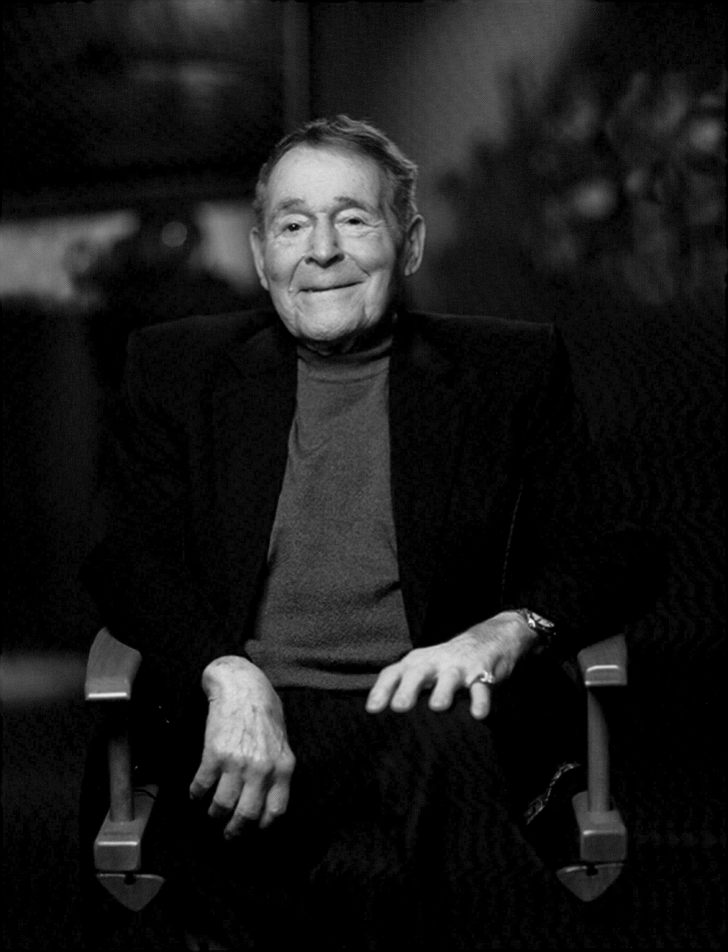

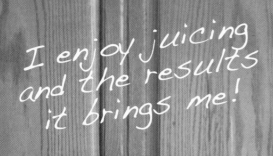

I enjoy juicing and the results it brings me!

CHAPTER FIFTEEN

Step 12: Consume Plenty of Fruits and Vegetables

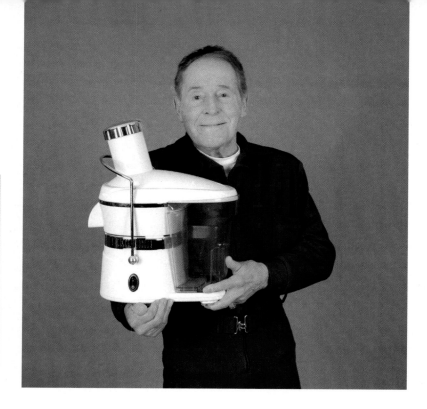

Juicing has been a regular part of my life since my late teens.

MY NUTRITIONAL PASSION: JUICING FOR HEALTH

Why the heck am I so enthusiastic about juicing? Is it because I sell the "Jack LaLanne Power Juicer"? Believe me, I get asked these questions. Frankly, I don't know if George Foreman uses his famous grill, or if Tiger Woods really prefers Nike. Does Anna Kournakova really wear Rolex watches? And what about Valerie Bertinelli – does she really follow Jenny Craig?

Who knows? What I do know is that juicing has been a regular part of my life since my late teens. But almost weekly someone asks me, "Jack, do you really juice? I see you on TV extolling the advantages of juicing …" My answer to all of you is a resounding yes! I love juicing and the results it brings me. The first juicer I ever owned was a press type. I had to grind up the fruits and vegetables first. It was so antiquated it was difficult to squeeze out all the juice. Ultimately a new generation of centrifugal juicers came on the market. I have owned most of them, including a huge commercial one that I was very proud of. It stood 20 inches high, measured 38 inches round and weighed a hefty 60 pounds. I still have it, in what I call my "museum memorabilia." I remember the first time Elaine ever came to my home. She was shocked at the size of this juicer in my kitchen. I juiced up some carrots and celery stalks and gave her a glass to taste. She loved it! She couldn't believe how sweet the juice tasted. She was well and truly switched on to juicing and still juices to this day.

Currently, with new technology, juicers have more powerful, high-output induction motors than ever before. No need to cut up your fruits and veggies. You get less noise and more juice. Technology has a way of keeping us up to date.

Before I started juicing I was a sugarholic. My love affair with ice cream and sodas actually made me sick. I got boils and pimples and the sugar destroyed the B vitamins and affected my brain, making me both hot tempered and confused. I got so sick I dropped out of school for six months.

Most Americans follow a diet of overprocessed, overcooked, often packaged foods. It seems to me that when man has his hand in processing or manufacturing foods, then many of the true nutrients are destroyed. Add to that food coloring, preservatives, sweeteners, ripening processes, chemicals of all kinds and you just know we are getting less than nature intended. I am of the firm belief that we eat too many overprocessed, cooked foods. It seems that almost everything we put in our body is cooked or grown and ripened artificially. Too much of this mucking about robs foods of their nourishment.

STEP
12

Giving your body the right food is like giving your car the right gas. Putting in anything other than the correct fuel will cause your automobile to splutter and die. In contrast, put raw and vital foods into your body and you will feel alive and energetic. Your body has some 80 trillion cells that are alive, and in my opinion if you put foodless, dead, processed, chemical-filled foods into your body you are not going to be properly nourished. This is why half the people you meet have no energy and feel tired all the time. Many even wake up tired.

You could ask, "Why not get your juice from a can or bottle from the store? It's too much trouble to get the juicer out, cut up the produce and to clean the appliance." Not with today's technology. Besides, when you juice the real McCoy you are getting the freshest product possible. Commercial juice normally contains preservatives, added sugar and salt, artificial flavoring and food coloring, and is often made of poor-quality produce that could no longer be sold. It goes against everything we get from juicing naturally.

Commercial juice is often made of poor-quality produce that could no longer be sold.

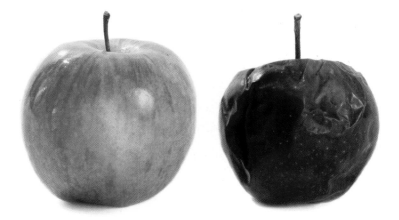

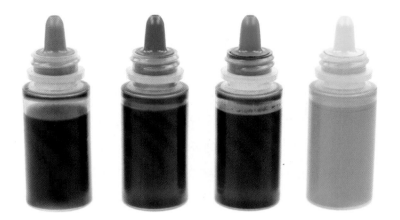

Can you think of anything more ridiculous than adding color to foods?

And talking about food coloring; can you imagine anything more ridiculous than adding color to meats, eggs, vegetables, drinks, fruits, you name it? Can't you just hear those directors sitting around a boardroom table? "I think we should add a little more yellow dye to outdo the competition. They've upped the yellow coloring in their eggs." "More red dye is needed in the raspberries. Sales are down." "Can we not make our meat sales stronger? Let's increase the volume of coloring." "Our soft drinks need more color. The public buy more when we supplement with orange."

Yes, it's madness. Where are we heading with this kind of thinking? Adding color to nature's foods to make them more appealing is ridiculous, and it's another example of the dumbing down of the North American people.

Juicing is not only a wonderful way to get nature's freshness into your body and hence to every cell in that body, it is also useful to those looking to lose weight. A glass of fresh juice helps to appease your appetite, so you don't want to eat as much. In addition it keeps your energy level up while making your taste buds dance with delight.

STEP
12

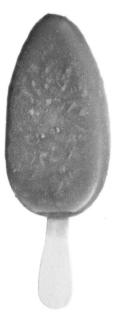

Make the youngsters frozen treats out of the juice. They'll love it!

Juicing is a way for us to be an example to our children. Too many of them are living on hot dogs, French fries, candy bars, ice cream and fast-food garbage. Why not get them juicing? Make the youngsters frozen treats out of the juice. They'll love it! You know how they love anything with a Popsicle stick.

To me, the best way to get 100 percent pure and natural vegetable and fruit juice into the body's enzyme network and thereby regulate and energize your body's organic functioning is to squeeze the juice directly from the source. Don't let it sit, because juice loses its natural nutrients as it sits around. And be warned. Store-bought juices may not be as pure or natural as you think. Read the label. Don't be surprised to discover that your juice is made from concentrated juices rather than fresh. Also, you may discover that filtered water and coloring have been added. Yes, that dastardly coloring returns yet again.

Fresh is best because to get enough vitamins, minerals and nutrients, your body needs to replace those lost on a daily basis. Nutritionists and the U.S.D.A. agree and advise that you eat 5 to 10 fresh fruits and vegetables a day. This is sound advice. Go back to your grocery store and walk down the canned and bottled juice aisle. How long do you think it's been since the actual apples, oranges or other fruit were picked? (And you can be pretty sure most were picked prior to ripening.)

The question often arises: Is organic better than non-organic? What's the difference? Organic or traditionally grown foods are grown without the use of chemical fertilizers and pesticides. Non-organic or conventionally grown fruits and vegetables may be grown using chemical fertilizers and pesticides. Produce sprayed

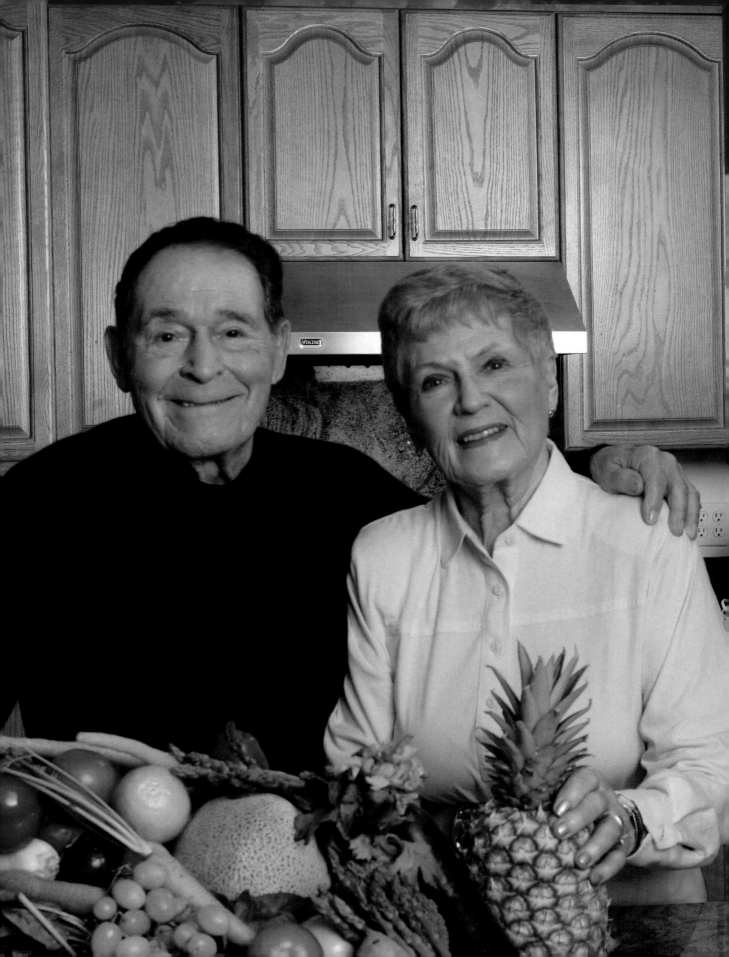

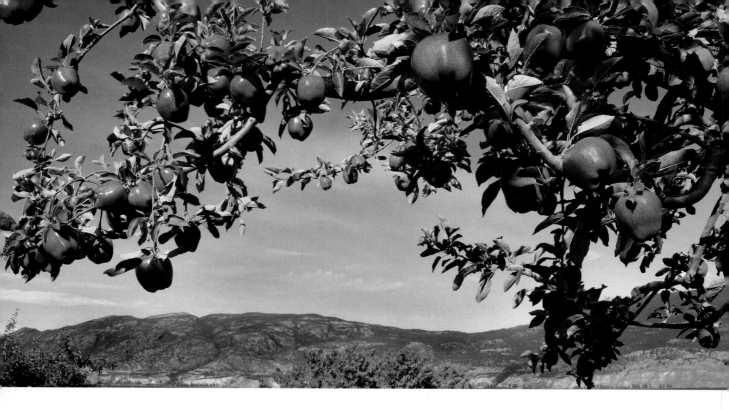

with chemicals is also usually picked unripe and then forcefully ripened upon arrival at its destination.

I maintain that you can smell the difference between organic and non-organic produce.

I maintain that you can smell the difference between organic and non-organic produce. An organic, or traditionally grown, apple may smell like an apple orchard in late summer, while a non-organic apple may have no smell at all. Ever tried the raspberries that come in those little square plastic containers? Notice their huge size, their unnatural bright redness and how completely tasteless they are. Compare that to organic farm-raised raspberries. Wow! They have a tangy fruit taste. Fruit that tastes like fruit. How novel in this day and age.

The fresher your fruit and vegetables, the richer they are in vitamins, minerals and other essential nutrients. Whether you choose to eat organic or non-organic produce it will still probably be superior to packaged, bottled, boxed or canned juices. Regardless of which fruit and vegetables you purchase to juice, be sure to wash them well before juicing.

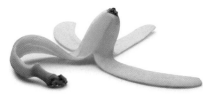

Some fruits and veggies cannot be juiced due to their inability to produce juice. Following is a list of foods you probably shouldn't try juicing. You can still enjoy the following products, of course, but don't put them in your juicer.

Avocados

You can add this healthy, high-fat veggie to your freshly blended juice. Remove the thick skin and center pit. Slice the avocado and place in the blender with your fresh juice.

Coconuts

Enormously difficult to juice. Like the avocado, the coconut is high in fat, so use sparingly. If you add coconut to your fresh juice it has to be added separately in the blender.

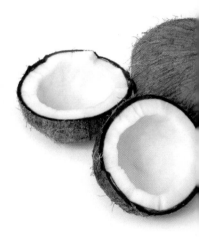

Bananas

There's no juice to be had, so don't put a banana in the juicer. Add it later in the blender. Bananas serve to thicken thin juices and are staples in making great-tasting creamy smoothies.

Leeks

Leeks do not lend themselves well to juicing. The outer layer is virtually impossible to juice. Be aware that if you do manage to juice leeks you will encounter a very potent juice that should be used sparingly.

Rhubarb

This vegetable is not a good candidate for juicing due to its oxalic acid content. Never use the green tops of rhubarb. The leaves contain toxins that can make you sick.

STEP
12

Juicing Tips

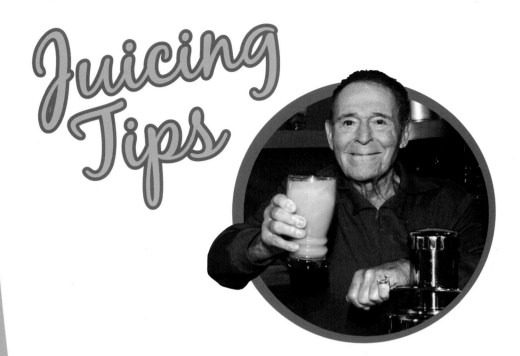

→ Enjoy your juice as soon as possible. Juice is at its best the second it's squeezed. Stir and drink up the minute it's done. It loses its potency over time.

→ If you have to store juice, use a glass jar with airtight lid. Place in the refrigerator. Make sure the glass jar is as full as possible. Any trapped air inside the jar will cause the juice to lose valuable nutrients.

→ You may add yogurt to thicken your juice. Use non-fat, non-sugar products though, especially if you are watching your weight.

→ Try to include the pith (the soft white layer between the fruit and the peel) when juicing citrus fruits. It contains lots of vitamins and minerals.

→ Citrus fruit peel is very bitter in taste and not good for juicing.

→ When juicing whole fruits or vegetables, make sure they are washed very thoroughly. Pay special attention to the navel area. Use a well-constructed brush. A colander may also be useful when washing fruits and veggies such as grapes, berries, Brussels sprouts, beans and mushrooms.

→ It's a good idea to let your family and friends in on the juicing process. Seeing their juices freshly made will make them feel truly special.

→ Adding vegetable and fruit pulp (the stuff that doesn't change into juice) to cooked dishes such as pasta sauce helps aid the digestive tract, as well as adding to your vitamin and mineral intake.

→ Drinking fresh juice before meals can curb your appetite, and consequently should support weight loss.

→ Substitute coffee in at least one of your breaks with a glass of juice. Your energy level will soar.

→ Cabbage doesn't refrigerate well. It takes on a foul smell. Otherwise you may refrigerate your juice if drinking it immediately is not an option, but bear in mind nutrients are lost during extended refrigeration.

→ If you want to make smoothies then a blender is necessary. Fruits and vegetables that shouldn't be put in a juicer (eg. bananas) can be added to juice in a blender for additional texture, taste and nutrition. Use a blender for smoothies, soups, frozen drinks, baby food and much more. A blender whips, chops and purees; these are functions a juicer cannot perform.

STEP
12

FRUITS

Most people enjoy fruits. That's good. However, most people don't eat much of it. Okay, they may have it in breakfast jam, or as a filling in pastries or apple pie, but the majority of people do not eat enough fresh fruits.

In the following dialogue I have listed some produce to be a "good source" of a nutrient, indicating that it offers at least 10 percent of the recommended daily intake per serving (raw), and those listed as an "excellent source" offer at least 20 percent of the recommended daily intake.

I refer to some produce as vegetable when in fact scientifically they belong in the fruit category. However, since these fruits i.e. tomatoes, zucchini and others, are commonly known as and referred to as vegetables I have listed them in the vegetable category so you can easily find them!

APPLES

Nutrients per 1 medium apple (182 g)

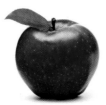

Good source of vitamin C, fiber, pectin, lutein and boron.

According to some experts, an improvement in memory is one of the benefits of eating apples on a regular basis, especially in the area of age-related memory loss. Others believe apples help keep your skin from wrinkling and may even promote hair growth on the scalp.

Apples are fat free, low in calories and a good source of fiber. The antioxidants in apples and other fruits and vegetables help ward off cardiovascular disease and cancer. Cholesterol levels may be lowered with the regular eating of apples, which are fairly inexpensive and available year round.

Protein	0 g	Potassium	195 mg	Niacin (B3)	0.2 mg
Fat	0 g	Vitamin A	98 IU	Vitamin B6	0.1 mg
Carbohydrate	25 g	Vitamin C	8 mg	Folate	5.5 mcg
Calcium	11 mg	Vitamin D	~	Vitamin B12	0 mcg
Phosphorus	20 mg	Vitamin E	0.3 mg	Pantothenic Acid	0.1 mg
Magnesium	9 mg	Vitamin K	~	Dietary Fiber	4 g
Iron	0 mg	Thiamin (B1)	0 mg	Kilojoules (kJ)	396
Sodium	2 mg	Riboflavin (B2)	0 mg	Calories	94

APRICOTS

Nutrients per 1 cup (155 g)

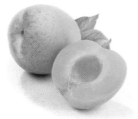

Excellent source of vitamin A, beta-carotene and vitamin C.
Good source of fiber and potassium.

Apricots are thought to keep the skin, hair, gums and various glands healthy, along with helping bones and teeth stay strong. The high vitamin A content helps fight infection by helping your immune system.

The fiber in apricots may help maintain blood-sugar levels in those who do not already have blood-sugar disorders such as diabetes, and it helps ease constipation, which in turn will likely reduce the risk of diverticulitis, colon cancer and hemorrhoids. Fiber-rich foods are usually low in calories.

Protein	2 g	Potassium	401 mg	Niacin (B3)	0.9 mg
Fat	0.6 g	Vitamin A	2985 IU	Vitamin B6	0.1 mg
Carbohydrate	17 g	Vitamin C	15.5 mg	Folate	13.9 mcg
Calcium	20 mg	Vitamin D	~	Vitamin B12	0 mcg
Phosphorus	36 mg	Vitamin E	1.4 mg	Pantothenic Acid	0.4 mg
Magnesium	16 mg	Vitamin K	5.1 mcg	Dietary Fiber	3 g
Iron	0.6 mg	Thiamin (B1)	0 mg	Kilojoules (kJ)	311
Sodium	2 mg	Riboflavin (B2)	0.1 mg	Calories	74

APRICOTS (DRIED)

Nutrients per 1 cup (130 g)

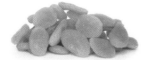

Excellent source of fiber, potassium, copper, vitamin A and magnesium.
Good source of iron, manganese and niacin.

Dried apricots are much higher in calories than fresh apricots and are an excellent source of the antioxidant beta-carotene. Dried fruits as a whole are more "nutrient-dense" than fresh fruit, however it's not only the fiber and minerals in the fruits that are concentrated. The carbohydrates (simple sugars) are also concentrated, hence the increase in calories. Dried apricots are always available and are a convenient and tasty way to include fiber, vitamin A and iron in your diet, but don't go overboard.

Protein	4.4 g	Potassium	1511 mg	Niacin (B3)	3.4 mg
Fat	0.7 g	Vitamin A	4686 IU	Vitamin B6	0.2 mg
Carbohydrate	81 g	Vitamin C	1.3 mg	Folate	13 mcg
Calcium	72 mg	Vitamin D	~	Vitamin B12	0 mcg
Phosphorus	92 mg	Vitamin E	5.6 mg	Pantothenic Acid	0.7 mg
Magnesium	41 mg	Vitamin K	4 mcg	Dietary Fiber	9 g
Iron	3 mg	Thiamin (B1)	0 mg	Kilojoules (kJ)	1310
Sodium	13 mg	Riboflavin (B2)	0.1 mg	Calories	313

BANANAS

Nutrients per 1 medium (118 g)

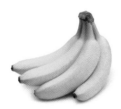

Excellent source of B6. Good source of potassium, vitamin C and manganese.

Bananas are essential to a super healthy diet. They have been traditionally used to settle the stomach, protect against acidity and even help to maintain the normal function of the heart. Bananas cannot be juiced, but they can be added to juice in a blender. They help make great smoothies. The natural sugars found in bananas make them a great energy source. The banana is one element of what doctors call the BRAT diet, i.e. bananas, rice, apples and toast. This diet is helpful for those who have a hard time digesting food because of illness or injury. People with an active lifestyle can benefit greatly from the potassium found in bananas.

Protein	1 g	Potassium	422 mg	Niacin (B3)	0.8 mg
Fat	0 g	Vitamin A	76 IU	Vitamin B6	0.4 mg
Carbohydrate	27 g	Vitamin C	10.3 mg	Folate	24 mcg
Calcium	6 mg	Vitamin D	~	Vitamin B12	0 mcg
Phosphorus	26 mg	Vitamin E	0.1 mg	Pantothenic Acid	0.4 mg
Magnesium	32 mg	Vitamin K	0.6 mcg	Dietary Fiber	3 g
Iron	0 mg	Thiamin (B1)	0 mg	Kilojoules (kJ)	440
Sodium	1 mg	Riboflavin (B2)	0.1 mg	Calories	105

BLACK CURRANTS

Nutrients per 1 cup (112 g)

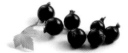

Excellent source of vitamin C.
Good source of potassium and manganese.

Black currants are available year round, with their peak season from May through August. They are an excellent source of vitamin C, which may be helpful in warding off colds in some people. Vitamin C is a water-soluble anti-oxidant vitamin capable of neutralizing potentially damaging free radicals. Also, vitamin C helps build white blood cells, which combat infection. This vitamin also helps heal wounds and maintain clear skin.

Protein	2 g	**Potassium**	361 mg	**Niacin (B3)**	0.3 mg
Fat	0 g	**Vitamin A**	258 IU	**Vitamin B6**	0.1 mg
Carbohydrate	17 g	**Vitamin C**	203 mg	**Folate**	~
Calcium	62 mg	**Vitamin D**	~	**Vitamin B12**	0 mcg
Phosphorus	66 mg	**Vitamin E**	1.1 mg	**Pantothenic Acid**	0.4 mg
Magnesium	27 mg	**Vitamin K**	~	**Dietary Fiber**	~
Iron	2 mg	**Thiamin (B1)**	0.1 mg	**Kilojoules (kJ)**	296
Sodium	2 mg	**Riboflavin (B2)**	0.1 mg	**Calories**	71

Vitamin C may be helpful in warding off colds in some people.

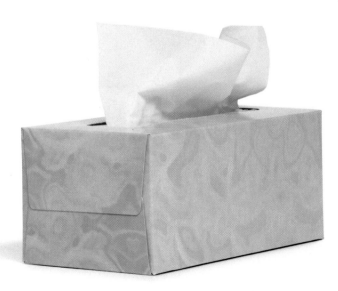

BLACKBERRIES

Nutrients per 1 cup (144 g)

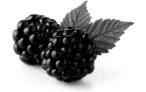

Excellent source of fiber, vitamin C and manganese.
Good source of potassium and copper.

The blackberry looks a lot like a raspberry, and has the same heavily seeded exterior, but its taste is milder. In the northwest U.S. and into Canada these berries grow practically everywhere. In fact they are so pervasive that residents seem to forget they are food and crazily leave this nutritious food to rot on the plant!

Vitamin C is a water-soluble vitamin and is required in order to build healthy tissue and support the immune system.

The jury is still out on some experts´ claim that potassium actually removes fluid from under the skin and puts it into the muscle.

Fiber helps maintain normal blood sugar levels in healthy people. It helps prevent occasional constipation and may be useful in reducing the risk of hemorrhoids and certain cancers.

Blackberries contain large numbers of antioxidants, which help prevent cancer, and flavonoids, which are known to improve heart health. This berry is available in season from May through August.

Protein	2 g	Potassium	233 mg	Niacin (B3)	0.9 mg
Fat	1 g	Vitamin A	308 IU	Vitamin B6	0 mg
Carbohydrate	14 g	Vitamin C	30 mg	Folate	36 mcg
Calcium	42 mg	Vitamin D	~	Vitamin B12	0 mcg
Phosphorus	32 mg	Vitamin E	1.7 mg	Pantothenic Acid	0.4 mg
Magnesium	29 mg	Vitamin K	28 mcg	Dietary Fiber	8 g
Iron	1 mg	Thiamin (B1)	0 mg	Kilojoules (kJ)	261
Sodium	1 mg	Riboflavin (B2)	0 mg	Calories	62

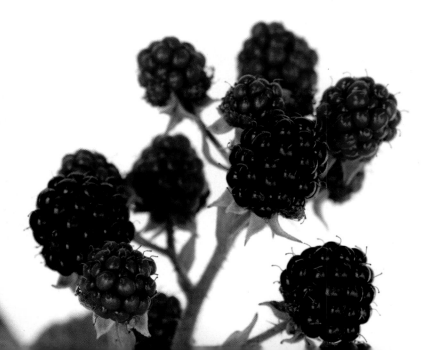

Blackberries contain large numbers of antioxidants, which help prevent cancer.

BLUEBERRIES

Nutrients per 1 cup (145 g)

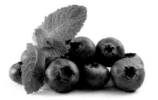

Excellent source of vitamin C, manganese and vitamin K. Good source of fiber.

I love blueberries. They taste delicious and are good news all the way. Blueberries contain more disease-fighting, age-proofing antioxidants than practically any other fruit or vegetable.

Blueberries, like other berries such as blackberries, contain ellagic acid, which is being studied to determine its anti-cancer properties. I am told the preliminary results have been encouraging. Also the Agriculture Research Service found that many berries, including blueberries, contain chemicals that may protect against cervical and breast cancer. Blueberries are grown in North America and are available in season from May to October. Wild blueberries have the best flavor.

Protein	1 g	Potassium	114 mg	Niacin (B3)	0.6 mg
Fat	0 g	Vitamin A	80 IU	Vitamin B6	0.1 mg
Carbohydrate	21 g	Vitamin C	14.4 mg	Folate	8.9 mcg
Calcium	9 mg	Vitamin D	~	Vitamin B12	0 mcg
Phosphorus	17 mg	Vitamin E	0.8 mg	Pantothenic Acid	0.2 mg
Magnesium	9 mg	Vitamin K	29 mcg	Dietary Fiber	3.6 g
Iron	0 mg	Thiamin (B1)	0.1 mg	Kilojoules (kJ)	353
Sodium	1 mg	Riboflavin (B2)	0.1 mg	Calories	84

CANTALOUPE MELON

Nutrients per 1 cup, diced (156 g)

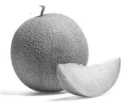

Excellent source of vitamins C and A. Good source of potassium.

Cantaloupe melons are a rich source of beta-carotene, which is converted to vitamin A in the body. This vitamin goes on to support healthy eyes and serves to keep bones, teeth, skin, hair, gums and various glands healthy.

Vitamin C goes a long way toward neutralizing potentially damaging free radicals. Vitamin C also supports white blood cells and is often required to heal bruises and open wounds.

Cantaloupe is grown in the U.S. While available year round, this melon is best in season from June to August.

Protein	1 g	Potassium	473 mg	Niacin (B3)	1.3 mg
Fat	0 g	Vitamin A	5987 IU	Vitamin B6	0.1 mg
Carbohydrate	16 g	Vitamin C	65 mg	Folate	37.2 mcg
Calcium	16 mg	Vitamin D	~	Vitamin B12	0 mcg
Phosphorus	26.5 mg	Vitamin E	0.1 mg	Pantothenic Acid	0.2 mg
Magnesium	21.2 mg	Vitamin K	4.4 mcg	Dietary Fiber	1.6 g
Iron	0 mg	Thiamin (B1)	0.1 mg	Kilojoules (kJ)	252
Sodium	28.3 mg	Riboflavin (B2)	0 mg	Calories	60

CHERRIES

Nutrients per 1 cup,
without pits (154 g)

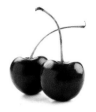

Good source of fiber and vitamin C.

Like many fruits, cherries are a good source of vitamin C, which among other important duties helps form collagen necessary for healthy skin. Cherries are also relatively high in the flavonoid quercetin, which is thought to reduce the risk of heart disease. Recent research is focusing on cherries for arthritis.

Cherries are one of the few known sources of melatonin, best known as a sleep enhancer and anti-aging agent that also possesses high antioxidant properties. Another compound in cherries is ellagic acid, which is currently being studied for possible cancer-preventing properties. Fresh cherries are available between June and August and are grown throughout the North American continent.

Protein	2 g	**Potassium**	342 mg	**Niacin (B3)**	0.2 mg
Fat	0 g	**Vitamin A**	98 IU	**Vitamin B6**	0.1 mg
Carbohydrate	23 g	**Vitamin C**	11 mg	**Folate**	6 mcg
Calcium	20 mg	**Vitamin D**	~	**Vitamin B12**	0 mcg
Phosphorus	32 mg	**Vitamin E**	0.1 mg	**Pantothenic Acid**	0.3 mg
Magnesium	17 mg	**Vitamin K**	3 mcg	**Dietary Fiber**	3 g
Iron	1 mg	**Thiamin (B1)**	0 mg	**Kilojoules (kJ)**	406
Sodium	0 mg	**Riboflavin (B2)**	0.1 mg	**Calories**	97

CRANBERRIES

Nutrients per 1 cup (110 g)

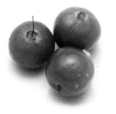

Excellent source of vitamin C. Good source of fiber and manganese.

Everyone should love cranberries. I do. Whereas you shouldn't rely on them above a doctor's advice, they have traditionally been used to help address urinary tract infections. Recent studies suggest that cranberries may be more beneficial to our health than previously thought. Preliminary studies have found cranberries may help prevent tooth decay, kidney stones and cancer. Also, they may help lower LDL (bad) cholesterol and raise HDL (good) cholesterol.

Cranberries are a little on the tart side in flavor. They do, however, juice well, and taste great when combined with grapes, strawberries, apples and peaches. Cranberries are available year round and are grown in the U.S., Canada and Europe.

Protein	0 g	**Potassium**	93 mg	**Niacin (B3)**	0.1 mg
Fat	0 g	**Vitamin A**	66 IU	**Vitamin B6**	0.1 mg
Carbohydrate	13 g	**Vitamin C**	15 mg	**Folate**	1.1 mcg
Calcium	9 mg	**Vitamin D**	~	**Vitamin B12**	0 mcg
Phosphorus	14 mg	**Vitamin E**	1.3 mg	**Pantothenic Acid**	0.3 mg
Magnesium	7 mg	**Vitamin K**	6 mcg	**Dietary Fiber**	5 g
Iron	0 mg	**Thiamin (B1)**	0 mg	**Kilojoules (kJ)**	212
Sodium	2 mg	**Riboflavin (B2)**	0 mg	**Calories**	50

FIGS

Nutrients per 2 large (128 g)

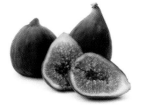

Good source of fiber.

Your digestive system works well only if it gets sufficient fiber on a regular basis. It certainly helps with the elimination process, which in turn may help reduce the risk of colon cancer and diverticular disease.

Those interested in controlling their weight would do well to include plenty of fiber in the diet. Amazingly, there are 150 varieties of figs. They are grown in the U.S. (California) and certain parts of Europe and Canada.

Important: Figs contain oxalates. Individuals who might have kidney or gall-bladder problems may want to avoid eating figs.

Protein	1 g	Potassium	298 mg	Niacin (B3)	0.6 mg
Fat	0.4 g	Vitamin A	182 IU	Vitamin B6	0.2 mg
Carbohydrate	24 g	Vitamin C	3 mg	Folate	7 mcg
Calcium	44 mg	Vitamin D	~	Vitamin B12	0 mcg
Phosphorus	18 mg	Vitamin E	0.2 mg	Pantothenic Acid	0.4 mg
Magnesium	22 mg	Vitamin K	6 mcg	Dietary Fiber	4 g
Iron	0.4 mg	Thiamin (B1)	0 mg	Kilojoules (kJ)	396
Sodium	1 mg	Riboflavin (B2)	0 mg	Calories	94

GRAPEFRUIT

Nutrients per half, large (166 g)

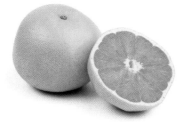

Excellent source of vitamins C and A.

Like other citrus fruits, grapefruit is chock full of vitamin C, a main ingredient in the fight against infection. Regular vitamin C intake helps you recover from workouts. In other words, it helps with muscle repair. Grapefruit interferes with some cholesterol medications, so check this with your pharmacist.

Nutrients called bioflavonoids, found in the white pith of citrus fruits, may be beneficial to the capillaries in pregnant women and may help heal minor bruising. Grapefruit is grown in the southern United States. Imported varieties are available year round but best between January and April, when it is in season.

Protein	1 g	Potassium	231 mg	Niacin (B3)	0.4 mg
Fat	0 g	Vitamin A	1539 IU	Vitamin B6	0.1 mg
Carbohydrate	13 g	Vitamin C	57 mg	Folate	16 mcg
Calcium	19 mg	Vitamin D	~	Vitamin B12	0 mcg
Phosphorus	13 mg	Vitamin E	0.2 mg	Pantothenic Acid	0.5 mg
Magnesium	13 mg	Vitamin K	0 mcg	Dietary Fiber	2 g
Iron	0 mg	Thiamin (B1)	0.1 mg	Kilojoules (kJ)	222
Sodium	0 mg	Riboflavin (B2)	0 mg	Calories	53

GRAPES

Nutrients per 1 cup,
red or green (151 g)

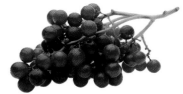

Excellent source of vitamins C and K.
Good source of copper. Also contains flavinoids, resveratrol, and tannins.

Believe it or not, there are literally thousands of varieties of grapes. They are used as a dessert, for a snack and in wine making.

Grapes are a heart-healthy fruit. The most nutritious are red grapes with seeds. They can be juiced with the seeds and the stems, since these sections contain valuable nutrients. The natural ingredients in grapes are thought to help with the risk of osteoporosis, bad cholesterol (LDL), blood clotting and urinary tract infections. They may also help protect arteries, thus enhancing cardiovascular function and promoting a healthy heart. The flavonoids in grapes may contribute greatly to the "healthy heart" tag that is universally claimed for grapes.

When grown in the northern hemisphere, grapes are in season from August to October. Grapes are grown throughout the world in temperate climates.

Tip: Elaine freezes grapes for a summer treat.

Protein	1 g	**Potassium**	288 mg	**Niacin (B3)**	0.3 mg
Fat	0 g	**Vitamin A**	100 IU	**Vitamin B6**	0.1 mg
Carbohydrate	27 g	**Vitamin C**	16 mg	**Folate**	3 mcg
Calcium	15 mg	**Vitamin D**	~	**Vitamin B12**	0 mcg
Phosphorus	30 mg	**Vitamin E**	0.3 mg	**Pantothenic Acid**	0.1 mg
Magnesium	11 mg	**Vitamin K**	22 mcg	**Dietary Fiber**	1 g
Iron	0.5 mg	**Thiamin (B1)**	0.1 mg	**Kilojoules (kJ)**	435
Sodium	3 mg	**Riboflavin (B2)**	0.1 mg	**Calories**	104

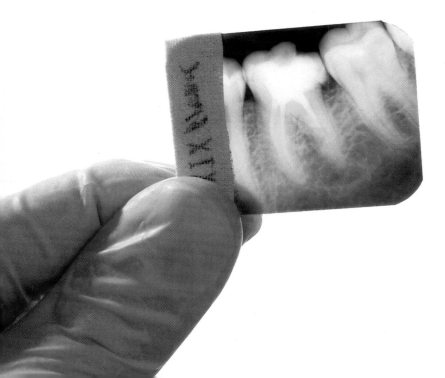

Vitamin A can help build strong teeth and bones, protect the eyes, and keep your skin, hair, gums, and numerous glands healthy.

There are literally thousands of varieties of grapes. Some are used in wine making.

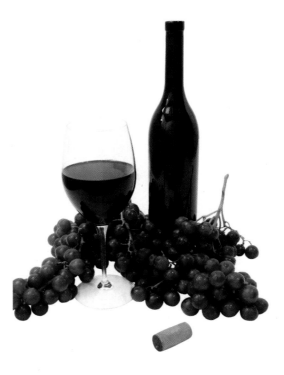

GUAVAS

Nutrients per 1 medium guava (55 g)

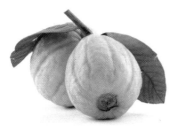

Excellent source of vitamin C. Good source of fiber and vitamin A.

Here we go again. Vitamin C hits the *excellent* rating. Vitamin C is a water-soluble antioxidant vitamin that neutralizes potentially damaging free radicals.

Guavas are also a good source of beta-carotene in the form of vitamin A. This vitamin serves a zillion requirements, such as building strong teeth and bones, protecting the eyes, and keeping the skin, hair, gums, and numerous glands healthy.

As a good source of fiber, this fruit helps regulate blood sugar in those without diabetes. Guavas come in different varieties. Some have seeds and others do not. It is important to remove the seeds beforehand if you are juicing. Fresh guava is available year round. In my opinion guava makes a great juice when combined with pineapples, mango, kiwi and strawberries. Guava is a tropical fruit that grows from the most southern areas of the U.S. to South America. In warmer regions, guava grows year round.

Protein	1 g	**Potassium**	229 mg	**Niacin (B3)**	0.6 mg
Fat	0.5 g	**Vitamin A**	343 IU	**Vitamin B6**	0.1 mg
Carbohydrate	8 g	**Vitamin C**	126 mg	**Folate**	27 mcg
Calcium	10 mg	**Vitamin D**	~	**Vitamin B12**	0 mcg
Phosphorus	22 mg	**Vitamin E**	0.4 mg	**Pantothenic Acid**	0.2 mg
Magnesium	12 mg	**Vitamin K**	1.4 mcg	**Dietary Fiber**	3 g
Iron	0 mg	**Thiamin (B1)**	0 mg	**Kilojoules (kJ)**	157
Sodium	1 mg	**Riboflavin (B2)**	0 mg	**Calories**	37

KIWI

Nutrients per 1 medium kiwi (76 g)

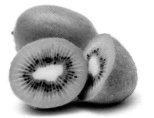

Excellent source of vitamins C and K.

Kiwi is packed with vitamin C, even more than you find in berries. Vitamin C actually helps the absorption of iron from plant sources. Women often have an iron deficiency.

Vitamin K is needed for blood clotting (handy when you accidentally cut yourself) and is especially good for the elderly in maintaining strong bones.

These tiny little fuzzy fruits can be juiced with the skin on and then joined by a juicier fruit such as pineapple, strawberries or apples.

Kiwi is grown in temperate regions throughout the world, and is available year round.

Protein	1 g	Potassium	237 mg	Niacin (B3)	0.3 mg
Fat	0 g	Vitamin A	66 IU	Vitamin B6	0 mg
Carbohydrate	11 g	Vitamin C	70 mg	Folate	19 mcg
Calcium	26 mg	Vitamin D	~	Vitamin B12	0 mcg
Phosphorus	26 mg	Vitamin E	1.1 mg	Pantothenic Acid	0.1 mg
Magnesium	13 mg	Vitamin K	31 mcg	Dietary Fiber	2 g
Iron	0 mg	Thiamin (B1)	0 mg	Kilojoules (kJ)	194
Sodium	2 mg	Riboflavin (B2)	0 mg	Calories	46

LEMON

Nutrients per 1 medium lemon (84 g)

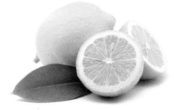

Excellent source of fiber and vitamin C. Good source of copper.

Very high in vitamin C, lemon wedges are frequently added to drinks of all kinds including water, to which it adds taste and nutrition. Lemons have a sour taste, and because of this they are best juiced together with less harsh fruits and vegetables.

Lemons (and limes) contain unique flavonoid compounds that have antioxidant properties and may have anti-cancer benefits. Other properties of the lemon may stop or retard cell division in many cancer cell lines. This fruit is also known for its antibiotic effects.

Lemons are grown in the U.S. and other warmer temperate regions and are available year round, but are best in season from December through February.

Protein	1 g	Potassium	116 mg	Niacin (B3)	0.1 mg
Fat	0 g	Vitamin A	19 IU	Vitamin B6	0.1 mg
Carbohydrate	78 g	Vitamin C	44 mg	Folate	9 mcg
Calcium	22 mg	Vitamin D	~	Vitamin B12	0 mcg
Phosphorus	13 mg	Vitamin E	0.1 mg	Pantothenic Acid	0.2 mg
Magnesium	7 mg	Vitamin K	0 mcg	Dietary Fiber	2 g
Iron	1 mg	Thiamin (B1)	0 mg	Kilojoules (kJ)	102
Sodium	2 mg	Riboflavin (B2)	0 mg	Calories	24

LIMES

Nutrients per 1 medium lime (67 g)

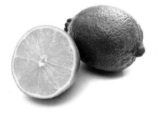

Excellent source of vitamin C.

Limes, like lemons, are often used as a garnish for drinks in bars and restaurants. The lime is a close cousin of the lemon. Vitamin C supports white blood cells, which combat infection, and this vitamin is essential for wound healing.

Limes are available throughout the year but are best in season from January through April. This fruit grows well in subtropical climates.

The slang term for a British citizen is "Limey." This term came about because English sailors discovered eating limes prevents scurvy, a disease that results from lack of vitamin C.

Protein	0 g	**Potassium**	68 mg	**Niacin (B3)**	0.1 mg
Fat	0 g	**Vitamin A**	34 IU	**Vitamin B6**	0 mg
Carbohydrate	7 g	**Vitamin C**	19 mg	**Folate**	5 mcg
Calcium	22 mg	**Vitamin D**	~	**Vitamin B12**	0 mcg
Phosphorus	12 mg	**Vitamin E**	0.1 mg	**Pantothenic Acid**	0.1 mg
Magnesium	4 mg	**Vitamin K**	0.4 mcg	**Dietary Fiber**	2 g
Iron	0 mg	**Thiamin (B1)**	0 mg	**Kilojoules (kJ)**	84
Sodium	1 mg	**Riboflavin (B2)**	0 mg	**Calories**	20

MANGOES

Nutrients per 1 cup, sliced (165 g)

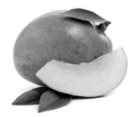

Excellent source of vitamins C and A.
Good source of fiber.

Mangoes are an excellent source of the antioxidant beta-carotene, which converts to vitamin A. This helps support the eyes and keep the skin, hair, gums, and various glands healthy. It also helps build strong bones and teeth. Vitamin A also helps strengthen the immune system.

Mangoes must be peeled and pitted before juicing. Follow with heavy juice-producing fruits such as pineapples or oranges to thin the thick mango nectar.

Mangoes are grown in tropical and sub-tropical regions, including the U.S. They are available year round but are best throughout late spring and summer.

Protein	0.8 g	**Potassium**	257 mg	**Niacin (B3)**	1 mg
Fat	0 g	**Vitamin A**	1262 IU	**Vitamin B6**	0.2 mg
Carbohydrate	28 g	**Vitamin C**	45 mg	**Folate**	23 mcg
Calcium	17 mg	**Vitamin D**	~	**Vitamin B12**	0 mcg
Phosphorus	18 mg	**Vitamin E**	1.8 mg	**Pantothenic Acid**	0.3 mg
Magnesium	15 mg	**Vitamin K**	7 mcg	**Dietary Fiber**	3 g
Iron	0 mg	**Thiamin (B1)**	0.1 mg	**Kilojoules (kJ)**	449
Sodium	3 mg	**Riboflavin (B2)**	0.1 mg	**Calories**	107

NECTARINES

Nutrients per 1 medium
nectarine (142 g)

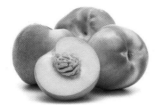

Good source of vitamin C.

The nectarine is closely related to the peach, but is slightly sweeter and does not have the fuzzy skin of the peach. Whatever you may have heard, nectarines are not the product of crossbreeding between a peach and a plum. Peaches and nectarines can be used interchangeably in recipes.

Nectarines contain a good serving of potassium, which is extremely beneficial to anyone with an active lifestyle. Bodybuilders and fitness athletes supplement with potassium to help take water from underneath the skin and throw it into the muscle.

This fruit is in season from May until September, but best in the summer. Imported varieties are available year round.

Protein	1 g	Potassium	285 mg	Niacin (B3)	1.6 mg
Fat	0 g	Vitamin A	471 IU	Vitamin B6	0 mg
Carbohydrate	15 g	Vitamin C	8 mg	Folate	7 mcg
Calcium	8 mg	Vitamin D	~	Vitamin B12	0 mcg
Phosphorus	36 mg	Vitamin E	1 mg	Pantothenic Acid	0.3 mg
Magnesium	13 mg	Vitamin K	3 mcg	Dietary Fiber	2 g
Iron	0 mg	Thiamin (B1)	0 mg	Kilojoules (kJ)	262
Sodium	0 mg	Riboflavin (B2)	0 mg	Calories	62

One of the most popular fruits in North America, oranges contain a great deal of vitamin C and no fat.

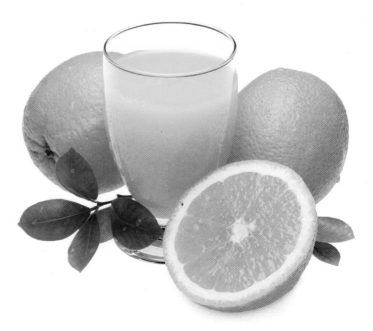

ORANGES

Nutrients per 1 medium
orange (131 g)

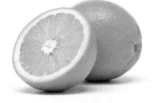

Excellent source of vitamin C. Good source of fiber, potassium, thiamin and folate.

Probably the most popular fruit in North America after apples, the orange contains a great deal of vitamin C and no fat.

Fiber may help reduce cholesterol levels. It also helps regulate blood sugar, and may reduce the likelihood of developing irritable bowel syndrome, cancer of the bowel and diverticulitis.

Beta-cryptoxanthin, an orange-red carotenoid, is found in oranges. Early studies have shown individuals consuming foods rich in beta-cryptoxanthin may have a reduced risk of developing lung cancer.

Oranges are grown in warm temperate parts of the world, including the southern U.S. and South Africa. They are available year round, but in North America they are best from January through March.

Protein	1 g	Potassium	237 mg	Niacin (B3)	0.4 mg
Fat	0 g	Vitamin A	295 IU	Vitamin B6	0.1 mg
Carbohydrate	15 g	Vitamin C	69 mg	Folate	40 mcg
Calcium	52 mg	Vitamin D	~	Vitamin B12	0 mcg
Phosphorus	18 mg	Vitamin E	0.2 mg	Pantothenic Acid	0.3 mg
Magnesium	13 mg	Vitamin K	0 mcg	Dietary Fiber	3 g
Iron	0 mg	Thiamin (B1)	0.1 mg	Kilojoules (kJ)	258
Sodium	0 mg	Riboflavin (B2)	0.1 mg	Calories	62

PAPAYA

Nutrients per 1 medium
papaya (304 g)

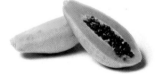

Excellent source of vitamin C, A, folate, potassium and fiber.

Papaya is a rich source of beta-carotene. It also contains papain and beta-crytoxanthin. Papain is an enzyme that is treasured by weight trainers, athletes and other vigorous exercisers because it helps you digest proteins, and muscle tissue is principally made up of proteins. If you are in need of bigger or more toned muscles, make papaya juice a part of your nutrition plan.

Papaya is grown in the U.S., Mexico, Puerto Rico and other tropical countries. It is available year round in quality grocery stores but best from June through September.

Protein	2 g	Potassium	781 mg	Niacin (B3)	1 mg
Fat	0 g	Vitamin A	3326 IU	Vitamin B6	0.1 mg
Carbohydrate	30 g	Vitamin C	188 mg	Folate	116 mcg
Calcium	73 mg	Vitamin D	~	Vitamin B12	0 mcg
Phosphorus	15 mg	Vitamin E	2 mg	Pantothenic Acid	0.7 mg
Magnesium	30 mg	Vitamin K	8 mcg	Dietary Fiber	5 g
Iron	0 mg	Thiamin (B1)	0.1 mg	Kilojoules (kJ)	498
Sodium	9 mg	Riboflavin (B2)	0.1 mg	Calories	119

PASSION FRUIT

Nutrients per 1 cup (236 g)

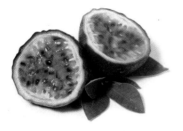

Excellent source of fiber, potassium, vitamins C and A. Good source of protein, iron, magnesium, phosphorus, copper, riboflavin, niacin and vitamin B6.

Fiber helps regulate blood-sugar levels, and can prevent and ease constipation. Modern research shows that this in turn may help reduce the risk of colon cancer and hemorrhoids, and may help with disorders like irritable bowel syndrome and diverticular disease.

Passion fruit is an good source of iron. Severe iron deficiency is associated with anemia, fatigue, weakness, loss of stamina, decreased ability to concentrate, infections, hair loss, dizziness, headaches, brittle nails, apathy and depression.

Magnesium deficiency may contribute to the likelihood of heart attack and strokes and can lead to osteoporosis. Minerals are needed in adequate numbers to ensure proper functioning of all bodily functions, including heart contraction.

Passion fruit can be enjoyed raw, seeds and all, but avoid eating the skin of the purple variety unless it's cooked. It's normally available year round.

Protein	5 g	Potassium	821 mg	Niacin (B3)	3 mg
Fat	2 g	Vitamin A	3002 IU	Vitamin B6	0.2 mg
Carbohydrate	55 g	Vitamin C	71 mg	Folate	33 mcg
Calcium	28 mg	Vitamin D	~	Vitamin B12	0 mcg
Phosphorus	160 mg	Vitamin E	0 mg	Pantothenic Acid	~
Magnesium	68 mg	Vitamin K	1.7 mcg	Dietary Fiber	24 g
Iron	4 mg	Thiamin (B1)	0 mg	Kilojoules (kJ)	959
Sodium	66 mg	Riboflavin (B2)	0.3 mg	Calories	229

Severe iron deficiency is associated with anemia, fatigue, weakness, loss of stamina, infections, hair loss, dizziness, headaches, apathy and depression.

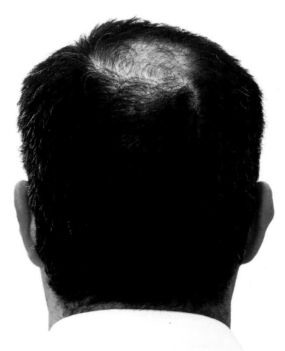

PEACH

Nutrients per 1 medium peach (150 g)

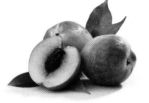

Good source of vitamin C.

Boy, do peaches taste great! You can juice them with the skin, but the pit has to be removed. Peaches are a good source of vitamin C and this is the most versatile vitamin of all. It is needed to form collagen for healthy skin and is essential in the formation of capillaries, bones and teeth. Vitamin C also helps the absorption of iron from plant sources. Deficiency in vitamin C can lead to broken veins, dry scalp, irritability, and weakness.

Domestic peaches are available from May to August and imported varieties are available year round.

Protein	1 g	Potassium	285 mg	Niacin (B3)	1.2 mg
Fat	0 g	Vitamin A	319 IU	Vitamin B6	0 mg
Carbohydrate	14 g	Vitamin C	10 mg	Folate	6 mcg
Calcium	9 mg	Vitamin D	~	Vitamin B12	0 mcg
Phosphorus	30 mg	Vitamin E	1 mg	Pantothenic Acid	0.2 mg
Magnesium	13 mg	Vitamin K	4 mcg	Dietary Fiber	2 g
Iron	0 mg	Thiamin (B1)	0 mg	Kilojoules (kJ)	245
Sodium	0 mg	Riboflavin (B2)	0 mg	Calories	58

PEARS

Nutrients per 1 medium pear (150 g)

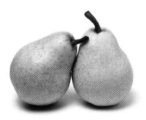

Excellent source of fiber. Good source of vitamin C.

Pears are both tasty and juicy, and the high concentration of fiber in pears helps regulate blood-sugar levels. Fiber, among other things, may have applications for promoting a healthy colon.

Few people realize that pears are closely related to the apple. There are literally thousands of varieties of pears including the Bosc, Bartlett, Anjou and Comice, all of which are grown in the U.S. and Canada.

Pears should be eaten or juiced with the skin intact, since the skin contains some of the fiber and other nutrients. Since there are so many varieties and since most of them store easily, pears are available year round, but most varieties are picked from July through September.

Protein	1 g	Potassium	285 mg	Niacin (B3)	1.2 mg
Fat	0 g	Vitamin A	489 IU	Vitamin B6	0 mg
Carbohydrate	15 g	Vitamin C	10 mg	Folate	6 mcg
Calcium	9 mg	Vitamin D	~	Vitamin B12	0 mcg
Phosphorus	30 mg	Vitamin E	1 mg	Pantothenic Acid	0.2 mg
Magnesium	13 mg	Vitamin K	4 mcg	Dietary Fiber	2 g
Iron	0 mg	Thiamin (B1)	0 mg	Kilojoules (kJ)	245
Sodium	0 mg	Riboflavin (B2)	0 mg	Calories	58

PINEAPPLE

Nutrients per 1 cup, diced (165 g)

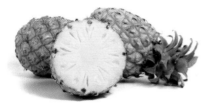

Excellent source of vitamin C and manganese.

Again the magic of vitamin C is up front and center in this juicy and delicious sweet fruit.

Manganese is a mineral element important in the breakdown of amino acids and the production of energy. It is necessary to metabolize vitamin B1 and vitamin E and activates numerous enzymes important for proper digestion and utilization of foods. Manganese keeps bones strong and healthy, helps your body break down fatty acids and cholesterol, helps maintain normal thyroid function, improves the health of your nerves and can protect your cells from free-radical damage.

Pineapple season runs from March through June. However, they are available year round in local markets. Try them on the grill!

Protein	1 g	**Potassium**	180 mg	**Niacin (B3)**	0.8 mg
Fat	0 g	**Vitamin A**	95 IU	**Vitamin B6**	0.2 mg
Carbohydrate	22 g	**Vitamin C**	78 mg	**Folate**	30 mcg
Calcium	21 mg	**Vitamin D**	~	**Vitamin B12**	0 mcg
Phosphorus	13 mg	**Vitamin E**	0 mg	**Pantothenic Acid**	0.4 mg
Magnesium	19 mg	**Vitamin K**	1.2 mcg	**Dietary Fiber**	2 g
Iron	0 mg	**Thiamin (B1)**	0.1 mg	**Kilojoules (kJ)**	345
Sodium	2 mg	**Riboflavin (B2)**	0.1 mg	**Calories**	82

PLUMS

Nutrients per 1 plum,
2-inch diameter (66 g)

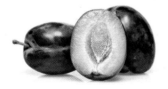

Good source of vitamin C.

Plums contain phenols (phytonutrients) that give them antioxidant properties. They are a relative of the peach and the nectarine.

Vitamin C is a water-soluble vitamin and is needed by the body to produce healthy skin and healthy tissue. It is also vitally important for a strong immune system. This versatile vitamin helps prevent the oxidation of cholesterol, thereby helping protect against heart disease.

Plums are available May through October.

Protein	0 g	**Potassium**	104 mg	**Niacin (B3)**	0.3 mg
Fat	0 g	**Vitamin A**	228 IU	**Vitamin B6**	0 mg
Carbohydrate	8 g	**Vitamin C**	6 mg	**Folate**	3 mcg
Calcium	4 mg	**Vitamin D**	~	**Vitamin B12**	0 mcg
Phosphorus	11 mg	**Vitamin E**	0.2 mg	**Pantothenic Acid**	0.1 mg
Magnesium	4 mg	**Vitamin K**	4 mcg	**Dietary Fiber**	1 g
Iron	0 mg	**Thiamin (B1)**	0 mg	**Kilojoules (kJ)**	127
Sodium	0 mg	**Riboflavin (B2)**	0 mg	**Calories**	30

POMEGRANATE

Nutrients per 1 medium
pomegranate (282 g)

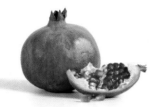

Good source of potassium and vitamin C.

The rind of the pomegranate is tough and dark red or brownish. Within the fruit are pockets of juicy, jewel-like fleshy seeds, which are edible. You can break open the pomegranate and work the seeds out of the inedible white, spongy membrane with your hands. Some stores now sell the "ariels"– how convenient!

Vitamin C is vital to the production of collagen, which is involved in the building and health of cartilage, joints, skin and blood vessels.

Pomegranates also contain flavonoids, which may help to lower the risk of certain cancers and reduce the risk of stroke and heart disease.

Fresh pomegranates are available between September and December.

Protein	5 g	Potassium	666 mg	Niacin (B3)	0.8 mg
Fat	3 g	Vitamin A	0 IU	Vitamin B6	0.2 mg
Carbohydrate	52 g	Vitamin C	28 mg	Folate	107 mcg
Calcium	28 mg	Vitamin D	~	Vitamin B12	0 mcg
Phosphorus	102 mg	Vitamin E	2 mg	Pantothenic Acid	1 mg
Magnesium	33 mg	Vitamin K	46 mcg	Dietary Fiber	11 g
Iron	1 mg	Thiamin (B1)	0.2 mg	Kilojoules (kJ)	980
Sodium	8 mg	Riboflavin (B2)	0.1 mg	Calories	234

Flavonoids may help to lower the risk of certain cancers and reduce the risk of stroke and heart disease.

PRUNES (DRIED PLUMS)

Nutrients per 1 cup, pitted (174 g)

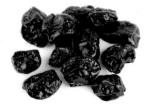

Excellent source of fiber, potassium, copper, manganese, niacin, vitamin B6 and vitamin A. Good source of phosphorus, thiamin, riboflavin and magnesium.

The reputation given to prunes is well earned. They are chock full of goodness. Prunes are in fact dried plums, and the drying process concentrates the nutrients (including the sugars and calories, so eat with prudence).

Prunes are an excellent source of vitamin A, in the form of beta-carotene, which acts as a fat-soluble antioxidant. Prunes may also help lower the risk of heart disease and colon cancer. The high amount of potassium helps regulate blood pressure and heart function. Potassium helps regulate water balance between the cells.

The soluble fiber in prunes helps stabilize blood-sugar levels, and helps reduce problems with the bowel, including constipation and associated diseases. It may also help reduce the risk of gastrointestinal problems and hemorrhoids.

Because they are dried, prunes are available year round.

Protein	4 g	Potassium	1274 mg	Niacin (B3)	3 mg
Fat	1 g	Vitamin A	1359 IU	Vitamin B6	0.4 mg
Carbohydrate	111 g	Vitamin C	1 mg	Folate	7 mcg
Calcium	74 mg	Vitamin D	~	Vitamin B12	0 mcg
Phosphorus	120 mg	Vitamin E	0.7 mg	Pantothenic Acid	0.7 mg
Magnesium	71 mg	Vitamin K	104 mcg	Dietary Fiber	12.4 g
Iron	1.6 mg	Thiamin (B1)	0.1 mg	Kilojoules (kJ)	1750
Sodium	3 mg	Riboflavin (B2)	0.3 mg	Calories	418

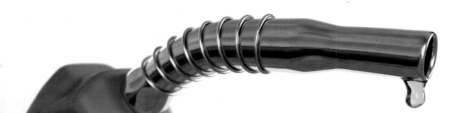

Giving your body the right food is like giving your car the right gas.

Juicing is a wonderful way to get nature's freshness into your body.

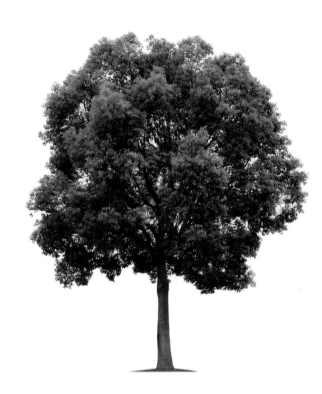

RASPBERRIES

Nutrients per 1 cup (123 g)

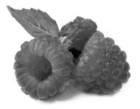

Excellent source of vitamin C, manganese, and fiber. Good source of vitamin K. Also contains ellagic acid and tannins, anthocyanins, and quercetin.

I call raspberries nature's nutritional powerhouses. They taste great too, especially if they are organically grown (grown without the use of pesticides and chemicals).

A recent preliminary study done on cultured cells by the Agriculture Research Service found: "Strawberries, blueberries and raspberries contain chemicals that may protect against cervical and breast cancer."

Grown in the U.S. and Canada, raspberries are in season from June through October.

Protein	1 g	**Potassium**	186 mg	**Niacin (B3)**	0.7 mg
Fat	1 g	**Vitamin A**	41 IU	**Vitamin B6**	0.1 mg
Carbohydrate	15 g	**Vitamin C**	32 mg	**Folate**	26 mcg
Calcium	31 mg	**Vitamin D**	~	**Vitamin B12**	0 mcg
Phosphorus	36 mg	**Vitamin E**	1 mg	**Pantothenic Acid**	0.4 mg
Magnesium	27 mg	**Vitamin K**	7 mcg	**Dietary Fiber**	8 g
Iron	0.8 mg	**Thiamin (B1)**	0 mg	**Kilojoules (kJ)**	268
Sodium	1 mg	**Riboflavin (B2)**	0 mg	**Calories**	64

STRAWBERRIES

Nutrients per 1 cup, whole (144 g)

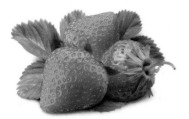

Excellent source of vitamin C and manganese. Good source of fiber.

Strawberries have a romantic connotation. Some feel a glass of champagne is not the same unless accompanied by a tiara of juicy ripe strawberries.

What I know for sure is that strawberries are a nutritional jewel, offering both fiber and vitamin C (more than any other berry) and manganese. Manganese is useful in maintaining a healthy nervous system. Vitamin C, a water-soluble vitamin, is needed for the body to produce healthy tissue. It is also important for a strong immune system and among other things helps prevent the oxidation of cholesterol, therefore helping protect against arteriosclerosis and diabetic heart disease. Inflammatory diseases too may be prevented with the use of vitamin C. Manganese is useful in maintaining a healthy nervous system.

Strawberries are grown almost everywhere temperate, from the gardens of England to the hills of California. Their short season runs from April to July, but they are available in stores year round.

Protein	1 g	Potassium	220 mg	Niacin (B3)	0.6 mg
Fat	0.43 g	Vitamin A	17 IU	Vitamin B6	0.1 mg
Carbohydrate	11 g	Vitamin C	84 mg	Folate	34 mcg
Calcium	23 mg	Vitamin D	~	Vitamin B12	0 mcg
Phosphorus	35 mg	Vitamin E	0.4 mg	Pantothenic Acid	0.2 mg
Magnesium	19 mg	Vitamin K	3 mcg	Dietary Fiber	3 g
Iron	0.6 mg	Thiamin (B1)	0 mg	Kilojoules (kJ)	196
Sodium	1 mg	Riboflavin (B2)	0 mg	Calories	46

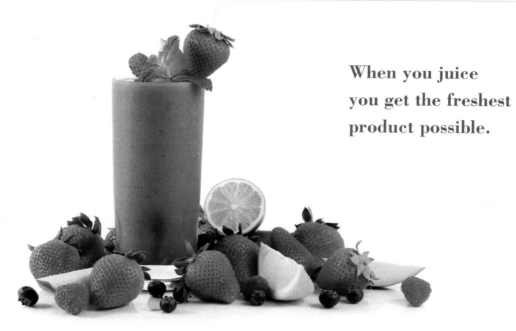

When you juice you get the freshest product possible.

> The fresher your fruit and vegetables, the richer they are in vitamins, minerals and other essential nutrients.

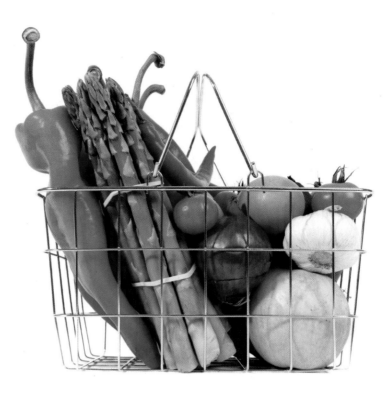

WATERMELONS

Nutrients per 1 cup, diced (152 g)

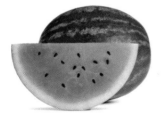

Excellent source of vitamin C. Good source of vitamin A.

Watermelons are extremely juicy (some say watery) fruits that can be very satisfying on a hot, humid day. They are an excellent source of the antioxidant beta-carotene, which is converted to vitamin A in the body. This helps support the eyes and keep the skin, hair, gums and various glands healthy. Vitamin A also helps bones and teeth and fights infection by contributing to a strong immune system.

Watermelons are an excellent source of vitamin C, a water-soluble vitamin capable of neutralizing potentially damaging free radicals.

Fresh watermelons are available in summer. They can be found in markets year round.

Protein	1 g	**Potassium**	170 mg	**Niacin (B3)**	0.3 mg
Fat	0 g	**Vitamin A**	865 IU	**Vitamin B6**	0.1 mg
Carbohydrate	11 g	**Vitamin C**	12 mg	**Folate**	5 mcg
Calcium	11 mg	**Vitamin D**	~	**Vitamin B12**	0 mcg
Phosphorus	17 mg	**Vitamin E**	0.1 mg	**Pantothenic Acid**	0.3 mg
Magnesium	15 mg	**Vitamin K**	0.2 mcg	**Dietary Fiber**	1 g
Iron	0.4 mg	**Thiamin (B1)**	0.1 mg	**Kilojoules (kJ)**	191
Sodium	2 mg	**Riboflavin (B2)**	0 mg	**Calories**	46

THE GLYCEMIC INDEX

Periodically, when high-protein, low-carb fad diets gain in popularity, carbohydrates get a bad rap. But carbs are essential for good health. The troubles come not simply from eating carbs, but rather when blood-sugar levels spike too high. This causes insulin overload, poor health and ultimately weight gain in those of us who can produce enough insulin, but for those of us with diabetes, these sugar spikes can spell disaster.

In 1981, Dr. David Jenkins and his team at the University of Toronto invented the Glycemic Index to demonstrate the speed at which specific foods raise blood-sugar levels. They conducted experiments to see how soon after eating a specific food the person displayed a blood-sugar spike, and the degree of the spike. Foods that produced a quick, high spike in blood sugar were given a high Glycemic Index (GI) rating, and those that produced slow, steady, longer-lasting blood-sugar elevations were given a low GI rating. Other foods fell in between.

And there were plenty of surprises. Some foods, such as a baked potato, that had been considered a great choice for slowly digested carbs, were shown to have a high GI, whereas some sweet fruits and other foods that had been previously thought a poor choice, such as grapes, were found to be quite low on the GI scale.

But you do not have to avoid all foods that have a high GI! Your body takes into account everything it's digesting at the same time. So if you combine high-GI foods, such as a baked potato, with low-GI foods, such as cottage cheese, then you will have successfully brought the GI down to a manageable level.

GLYCEMIC INDEX (GI) FOOD CHART

CEREALS

Low GI (Under 55)		Medium GI (56-69)		High GI (70+)	
Kellogg's All Bran	51	Shredded Wheat	67	Kellogg's Cornflakes	84
Kellogg's Bran Buds	45	Quaker Puffed Wheat	67	Kellogg's Rice Krispies	82
Kellogg's Special K	54				
Oatmeal	49				

GRAINS

Low GI (Under 55)		Medium GI (56-69)		High GI (70+)	
Buckwheat	54	Basmati Rice	58	Short-grain White Rice	72
Bulgur	48	Long-grain White Rice	56		
Brown Rice	55	Taco Shells	68		

FRUIT

Low GI (Under 55)		Medium GI (56-69)		High GI (70+)	
Apple	38	Cantaloupe	65	Watermelon	103
Banana	55	Papaya	58		
Cherries	22	Pineapple	66		
Grapefruit	25				
Grapes	46				
Kiwi	52				
Mango	55				
Orange	44				
Pear	38				
Plum	39				

Fruit sometimes gets a bad rap, but you can tell by this chart that fruits are a great choice.

VEGETABLES					
Low GI (Under 55)		**Medium GI (56-69)**		**High GI (70+)**	
Broccoli	10	Beets	69	Parsnips	97
Cabbage	10	Potato (new)	62	Potato (baked)	93
Carrots	49			Potato (mashed)	86
Corn	55			Potato (instant)	86
Green Peas	48			Potato (french fries)	75
Lettuce	10			Pumpkin	75
Mushrooms	10				
Onions	10				
Red Peppers	10				
Sweet Potato	54				

BEANS					
Low GI (Under 55)		**Medium GI (56-69)**		**High GI (70+)**	
Baked Beans	48			Broad Beans	79
Cannellini Beans	31				
Garbanzo Beans (Chickpeas)	33				
Lentils	30				
Lima Beans	32				
Navy Beans	38				
Pinto Beans	39				
Red Kidney Beans	27				
Soy Beans	18				
White Beans	31				

Beans are always recommended to keep blood-sugar levels stable, and here you can see why.

PASTA		
Low GI (Under 55)	**Medium GI (56-69)**	**High GI (70+)**
Spaghetti 43	Rice vermicelli 58	
Ravioli (meat) 39		
Fettuccini (egg) 32		
Spiral Pasta 43		
Capellini 45		
Linguine 46		
Macaroni 47		

Whole-grain pasta is the best choice.

BREADS (including Muffins and Cakes)		
Low GI (Under 55)	**Medium GI (56-69)**	**High GI (70+)**
Pumpernickel Bread 51	Blueberry Muffin 59	Bagel 72
Sourdough Bread 52	Croissant 67	Donut 76
Sponge Cake 46	Pita Bread 57	Rye Bread 76
Whole-Wheat Bread	Whole-Wheat Bread 69	Waffles 76
(Stone-Ground) 53		White Bread 70

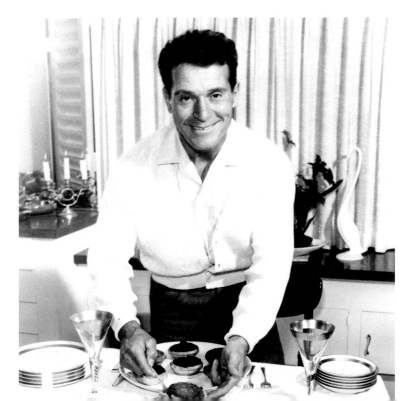

DAIRY		
Low GI (Under 55)	**Medium GI (56-69)**	**High GI (70+)**
Milk (whole) 22	Ice Cream (whole) 61	
Milk (skimmed) 32		
Milk (chocolate) 34		
Yogurt (low-fat) 33		

SNACKS		
Low GI (Under 55)	**Medium GI (56-69)**	**High GI (70+)**
Cashews 22		Corn Chips 72
Peanuts 14		Jelly Beans 80
Popcorn 55		Pretzels 83
Walnuts 15		

The type of snack you choose makes a huge difference!

CRACKERS and CRISPBREAD		
Low GI (Under 55)	**Medium GI (56-69)**	**High GI (70+)**
	Ryvita Crispbread 69	Graham Crackers 74
	Stoned Wheat Thins 67	Kavli Crispbread 71
		Melba Toast 70
		Rice Cakes 82
		Rice Crackers 91
		Soda Crackers 74
		Water Crackers 78

Crackers are not the best choice for health. Make sure to combine them with some slow-digesting protein.

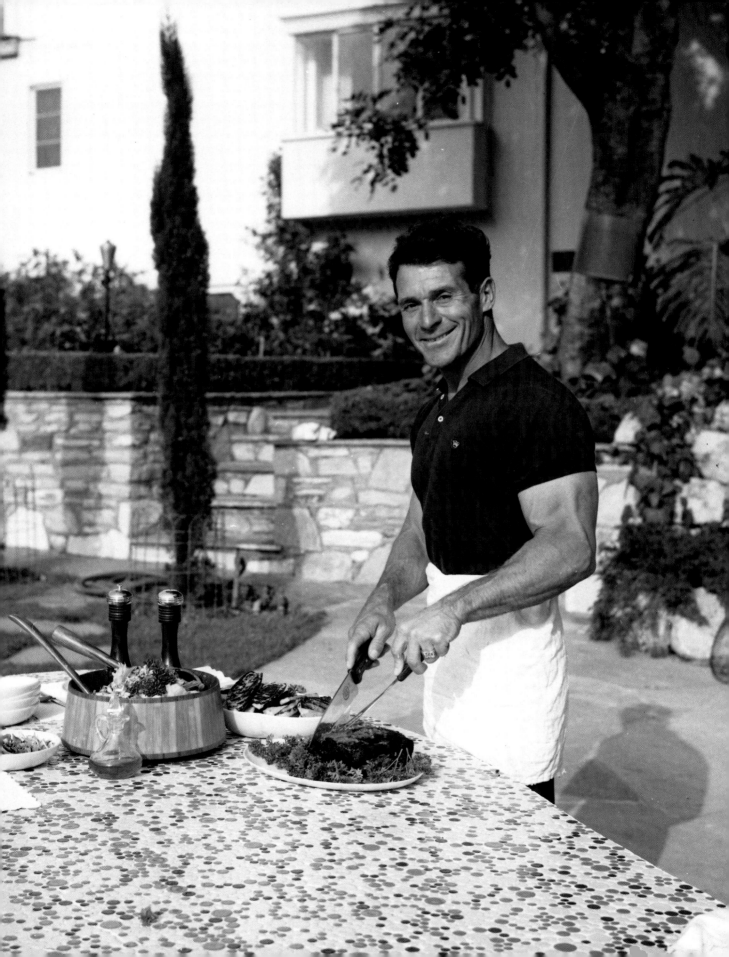

VEGETABLES

For the purpose of this section I have designated vegetables as a "good source" of a specific nutrient if they contain at least 10 percent of the daily recommended intake of that nutrient. Vegetables considered an "excellent source" of a specific nutrient contain at least 20 percent of the daily recommended intake. These calculations are based on USDA analysis of fruits and vegetables.

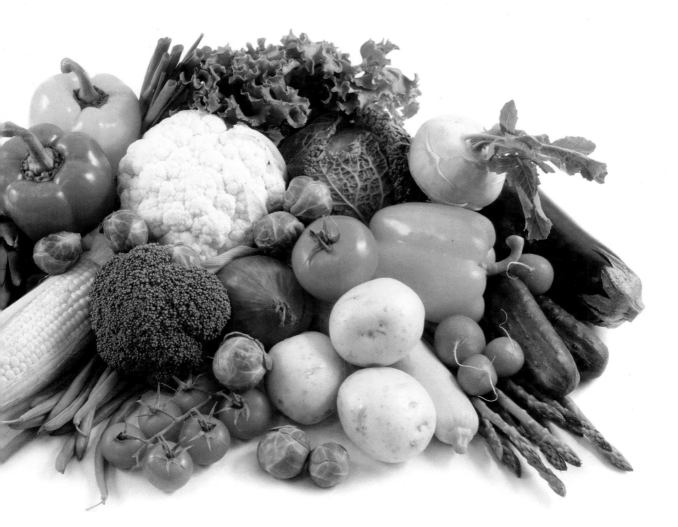

ARTICHOKES

Nutrients per 1 medium (128 g)

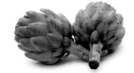

Excellent source of vitamin C, fiber, folate and vitamin K.

Good source of magnesium, potassium, manganese, phosphorus and copper.

Deficiencies of vitamin C may cause increased bruising. Vitamin C is also associated with anti-inflammatory properties that may inhibit the development of asthmatic symptoms. Potassium in artichokes help reduce urinary calcium excretion, and this appears to lower the risk of kidney stones.

Artichokes are available year round but are best at their peak season between March and May.

Protein	4 g	Potassium	474 mg	Niacin (B3)	1.3 mg
Fat	0 g	Vitamin A	17 IU	Vitamin B6	0.1 mg
Carbohydrate	13 g	Vitamin C	15 mg	Folate	87 mcg
Calcium	56 mg	Vitamin D	~	Vitamin B12	0 mcg
Phosphorus	115 mg	Vitamin E	0.2 mg	Pantothenic Acid	0.4 mg
Magnesium	77 mg	Vitamin K	19 mcg	Dietary Fiber	7 g
Iron	1.6 mg	Thiamin (B1)	0.1 mg	Kilojoules (kJ)	251
Sodium	120 mg	Riboflavin (B2)	0.1 mg	Calories	60

ASPARAGUS

Nutrients per 1 cup (134 g)

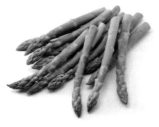

Tip: Asparagus grills nicely.

Good source of vitamin C, folate (folic acid) and vitamin K.

Folate, or folic acid, comes from nature's plants. Scientific studies have indicated that increasing your consumption of folic acid before and during pregnancy may help prevent neural-tube birth defects such as spina bifida, which can prove deadly in some cases. You can also improve your cardiovascular system by consuming enough folic acid. Perhaps more relevant if you're older is that folic acid is thought to help prevent both Alzheimer's and Parkinson's diseases, and to help prevent dementia of all kinds.

Those who suffer from edema and other problems with swelling are traditionally prescribed an asparagus-rich diet because this vegetable has diuretic properties.

Asparagus comes in green, white and purple varieties. Its peak season is from February through June, but as with most produce, it is available year round.

Protein	3 g	Potassium	271 mg	Niacin (B3)	1.3 mg
Fat	0.16 g	Vitamin A	1013 IU	Vitamin B6	0.1 mg
Carbohydrate	5 g	Vitamin C	7 mg	Folate	69 mcg
Calcium	32 mg	Vitamin D	~	Vitamin B12	0 mcg
Phosphorus	70 mg	Vitamin E	1.5 mg	Pantothenic Acid	0.4 mg
Magnesium	19 mg	Vitamin K	56 mcg	Dietary Fiber	3 g
Iron	2.9 mg	Thiamin (B1)	0.2 mg	Kilojoules (kJ)	112
Sodium	3 mg	Riboflavin (B2)	0.2 mg	Calories	27

AVOCADO

Nutrients per 1 cup, sliced (146 g)

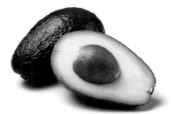

Excellent source of dietary fiber, potassium, vitamin C, vitamin K, folate and pantothenic acid (B5).

Good source of magnesium, copper, manganese, riboflavin and niacin (B3).

Of course this advice does not replace that of your medical practitioner, but eating avocados helps you decrease your cholesterol levels. Consumption of this food might also help such circulatory conditions as high blood pressure, heart disease and stroke.

The avocado is high in fat, but it's good fat. The most popular avocados in the U.S. are the HAAS variety, although other types are available from Mexico, Guatemala and the West Indies. The edible portion of the avocado is the soft, yellow green flesh. The skin and pit are inedible.

Protein	3 g	**Potassium**	708 mg	**Niacin (B3)**	2.5 mg
Fat	21 g	**Vitamin A**	213 IU	**Vitamin B6**	0.4 mg
Carbohydrate	12 g	**Vitamin C**	15 mg	**Folate**	118 mcg
Calcium	18 mg	**Vitamin D**	~	**Vitamin B12**	0.1 mcg
Phosphorus	76 mg	**Vitamin E**	3 mg	**Pantothenic Acid**	2 mg
Magnesium	42 mg	**Vitamin K**	30 mcg	**Dietary Fiber**	9 g
Iron	0.8 mg	**Thiamin (B1)**	0.2 mg	**Kilojoules (kJ)**	980
Sodium	10 mg	**Riboflavin (B2)**	0.2 mg	**Calories**	234

BEETS

Nutrients per 1 cup (136 g)

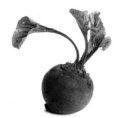

Excellent source of folate.

Good source of potassium, fiber, manganese and vitamin C.

Of all veggies beets have the highest sugar content, yet they are comparatively low in calories. The beet is powerful in that its nutrients are considered good for cleansing the kidneys and may help form a safeguard against some forms of cancer.

When you juice beets you get one heck of a health food delivery. Beet greens are also edible and are a good source of vitamin C and vitamin A.

Fresh beets are grown in most areas of Canada and the U.S., and crops are harvested throughout the year. Peak months are June through October.

Protein	2 g	**Potassium**	442 mg	**Niacin (B3)**	0.5 mg
Fat	0.23 g	**Vitamin A**	45 IU	**Vitamin B6**	0.1 mg
Carbohydrate	13 g	**Vitamin C**	7 mg	**Folate**	148 mcg
Calcium	22 mg	**Vitamin D**	~	**Vitamin B12**	0 mcg
Phosphorus	54 mg	**Vitamin E**	0.1 mg	**Pantothenic Acid**	0.2 mg
Magnesium	31 mg	**Vitamin K**	0.3 mcg	**Dietary Fiber**	4 g
Iron	1.1 mg	**Thiamin (B1)**	0 mg	**Kilojoules (kJ)**	245
Sodium	106 mg	**Riboflavin (B2)**	0.1 mg	**Calories**	58

BROCCOLI

Nutrients per 1 cup, chopped (91 g)

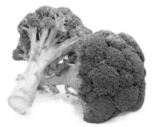

Excellent source of vitamin K and vitamin C. Good source of vitamin A and folate.

Photochemicals sulforahane and indoles are found in broccoli. Studies have shown that indule-3-carbinol is a breakdown product that may help to reduce the risk of cancer. In addition this product may inhibit the growth of breast cancer cells. Research has shown that by eating broccoli regularly you may have a lesser chance of developing cataracts.

Vitamin C helps the body absorb calcium, which is important for the formation of strong bones. Broccoli may also be an immune-system booster. Broccoli is a good source of folic acid, which helps prevent heart disease, Parkinson's and dementia. Broccoli can be eaten raw or cooked. It is available year round.

Protein	3 g	Potassium	288 mg	Niacin (B3)	0.6 mg
Fat	0 g	Vitamin A	567 IU	Vitamin B6	0.2 mg
Carbohydrate	6 g	Vitamin C	81 mg	Folate	57 mcg
Calcium	42 mg	Vitamin D	~	Vitamin B12	0 mcg
Phosphorus	60 mg	Vitamin E	0.7 mg	Pantothenic Acid	0.5 mg
Magnesium	19 mg	Vitamin K	93 mcg	Dietary Fiber	2.4 g
Iron	0.7 mg	Thiamin (B1)	0.1 mg	Kilojoules (kJ)	129
Sodium	30 mg	Riboflavin (B2)	0.1 mg	Calories	31

BRUSSELS SPROUTS

Nutrients per 1 cup (88 g)

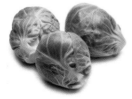

Excellent source of vitamin K and vitamin C. Good source of vitamin A, folate and fiber.

Brussels sprouts deliver important dosages of vitamin C, which strongly supports the immune system and also manufactures collagen. Collagen is the protein that takes care of skin and the connective tissue, cartilage and tendons. There is conjecture that this may reduce the risk of heart attacks, stroke and cancer.

Folate is found in large measure in Brussels sprouts. Folic-acid deficiency can cause everything from birth defects to heart disease to dementia.

Colon health is supported by the fiber content in Brussels sprouts. Brussels sprouts are available year round in North America.

Protein	3 g	Potassium	342 mg	Niacin (B3)	0.7 mg
Fat	0 g	Vitamin A	664 IU	Vitamin B6	0.2 mg
Carbohydrate	8 g	Vitamin C	75 mg	Folate	54 mcg
Calcium	37 mg	Vitamin D	~	Vitamin B12	0 mcg
Phosphorus	61 mg	Vitamin E	0.8 mg	Pantothenic Acid	0.3 mg
Magnesium	20 mg	Vitamin K	156 mcg	Dietary Fiber	3 g
Iron	1.2 mg	Thiamin (B1)	0.1 mg	Kilojoules (kJ)	158
Sodium	22 mg	Riboflavin (B2)	0.1 mg	Calories	38

CABBAGE

Nutrients per 1 cup, chopped (89 g)

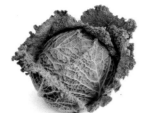

Excellent source of vitamins K and C.
Good source of manganese.

Cabbage contains the photochemicals sulforahane and indoles. Indole-3-carbinol is a breakdown product found in cruciferous vegetables. This substance is thought to reduce the risk of cancer but research is not conclusive.

Cabbage consumption is suspected to decrease the risk of cataracts. Raw cabbage juice has been used as an effective treatment for peptic ulcers. Cabbage comes in three major types: green, red and savoy. These vegetables are available year round with a late-fall early-winter peak.

Protein	1 g	Potassium	151 mg	Niacin (B3)	0.2 mg
Fat	0 g	Vitamin A	87 IU	Vitamin B6	0.1 mg
Carbohydrate	5 g	Vitamin C	33 mg	Folate	38 mcg
Calcium	35 mg	Vitamin D	~	Vitamin B12	0 mcg
Phosphorus	23 mg	Vitamin E	0.1 mg	Pantothenic Acid	0.2 mg
Magnesium	11 mg	Vitamin K	68 mcg	Dietary Fiber	2 g
Iron	0.4 mg	Thiamin (B1)	0.1 mg	Kilojoules (kJ)	93
Sodium	16 mg	Riboflavin (B2)	0 mg	Calories	22

CARROTS

Nutrients per 1 medium (61 g)

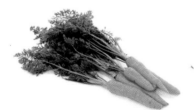
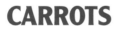

Excellent source of vitamin A. Good source of fiber, vitamin C, vitamin B6, potassium, vitamin B1, vitamin B3, phosphorus, vitamin B2, vitamin B5 and vitamin K.

You can't beat carrots as a solid source of good nutrition. Not only are the calories low but the taste is great. They make an excellent snack food for children or adults. Because carrots have a high beta-carotene content they may help to reduce the risk of coronary heart disease and several kinds of cancer.

Energy levels increase when one takes a lot of beta-carotene. In addition beta-carotene in carrots may help us reduce the risk of poor night vision and vitamin A may help prevent retinitis pigment.

Carrots are found in a variety of colors: white, red, yellow and purple, but the most common variety is orange. They are widely available all year round.

Protein	1 g	Potassium	195 mg	Niacin (B3)	0.6 mg
Fat	0 g	Vitamin A	10190 IU	Vitamin B6	0.1 mg
Carbohydrate	6 g	Vitamin C	4 mg	Folate	12 mcg
Calcium	20 mg	Vitamin D	~	Vitamin B12	0 mcg
Phosphorus	21 mg	Vitamin E	0.4 mg	Pantothenic Acid	0.2 mg
Magnesium	7 mg	Vitamin K	8 mcg	Dietary Fiber	2 g
Iron	0.2 mg	Thiamin (B1)	0 mg	Kilojoules (kJ)	105
Sodium	42 mg	Riboflavin (B2)	0 mg	Calories	25

CAULIFLOWER

Nutrients per 1 cup (100g)

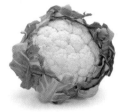

Excellent source of vitamin K and vitamin C.
Good source of folate and fiber.

The phytochemicals sulforaphane and indoles are present in cauliflower. Eating this vegetable often can help prevent cancer. Cauliflower may also have some antioxidant functions. Some researchers feel that vegetables in the carotenoid family, of which cauliflower is a member, may help prevent cataracts.

The vitamin C in cauliflower helps the body absorb calcium, which is important for strong bones. People with untreated thyroid problems may want to consult their doctor before eating cauliflower. Goitrogens found naturally in cauliflower could interfere with thyroid function.

Protein	2 g	Potassium	303 mg	Niacin (B3)	0.5 mg
Fat	0 g	Vitamin A	13 IU	Vitamin B6	0.2 mg
Carbohydrate	5 g	Vitamin C	46 mg	Folate	57 mcg
Calcium	22 mg	Vitamin D	~	Vitamin B12	0 mcg
Phosphorus	44 mg	Vitamin E	0.1 mg	Pantothenic Acid	0.7 mg
Magnesium	15 mg	Vitamin K	16 mcg	Dietary Fiber	3 g
Iron	0.4 mg	Thiamin (B1)	0.1 mg	Kilojoules (kJ)	105
Sodium	30 mg	Riboflavin (B2)	0.1 mg	Calories	25

CELERY

Nutrients per 1 stalk (40 g)

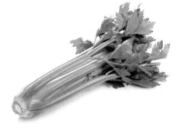

Good source of vitamin A and vitamin K.

Celery is an amazing no-fat, low-calorie vegetable. Dieters favor celery because it contains compounds that promote health, and helps keep weight in check. Children should be encouraged to chew on celery sticks rather than candy or chocolate bars. Add some natural peanut butter for healthy fat.

Folate (folic acid) contributes to the maintenance of new cells, and helps to reduce the risk of cardiovascular disease, dementia, Parkinson's disease and certain cancers. Folate is also recommended for pregnant women before and during pregnancy to reduce the risk of neural birth defects.

Vitamin K is known to improve the blood's clotting ability and vitamin A helps mucous membranes, skin and hair.

Protein	0 g	Potassium	104 mg	Niacin (B3)	0.1 mg
Fat	0 g	Vitamin A	180 IU	Vitamin B6	0 mg
Carbohydrate	1 g	Vitamin C	1.2 mg	Folate	14 mcg
Calcium	16 mg	Vitamin D	~	Vitamin B12	0 mcg
Phosphorus	10 mg	Vitamin E	0.1 mg	Pantothenic Acid	0.1 mg
Magnesium	4 mg	Vitamin K	12 mcg	Dietary Fiber	1 g
Iron	0.1 mg	Thiamin (B1)	0 mg	Kilojoules (kJ)	26
Sodium	32 mg	Riboflavin (B2)	0 mg	Calories	6

COLLARD GREENS

Nutrients per 1 cup, chopped (36g)

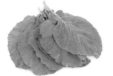

Excellent course of vitamins C, A (in the form of beta-carotene) and E.

Vitamin A is vital to a strong immune system, mucous membranes, skin and hair. Collard greens are rich in phytonutrients and, according to some non-conclusive research, may help reduce the risk of some cancers.

Vitamin C is the primary water-soluble antioxidant in the body, and may reduce the risk of some cancers and heart disease.

Collard greens are among the small number of vegetables that contain minute amounts of oxalates, so those with existing and potential kidney or gall-bladder problems may want to avoid eating collard greens.

Protein	0.88 g	Potassium	61 mg	Niacin (B3)	0.267 mg
Fat	0.15 g	Vitamin A	2400 IU	Vitamin B6	0.1 mg
Carbohydrate	2.05 g	Vitamin C	12.7 mg	Folate	59.8 mcg
Calcium	52 mg	Vitamin D	~	Vitamin B12	~
Phosphorus	4 mg	Vitamin E	0.8 mg	Pantothenic Acid	0.1 mg
Magnesium	3 mg	Vitamin K	184 mcg	Dietary Fiber	1 g
Iron	0.1 mg	Thiamin (B1)	0.19 mg	Kilojoules (kJ)	45
Sodium	7 mg	Riboflavin (B2)	0.047 mg	Calories	11

CUCUMBER

Nutrients per 1 cucumber, 8 1/4 inches long (300 g)

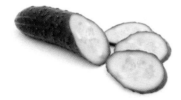

Excellent source of vitamin K. Good source of potassium, manganese and vitamin C.

There's no fat in cucumbers and they have a very high quantity of water. For ages we have placed cucumber slices on our faces to hydrate the skin and improve the complexion. You can help reduce puffiness under the eyes and soothe a sunburn in this way. The silica in cucumbers helps keep muscles, tendons, ligaments and cartilage healthy.

Vitamin K helps blood to clot and builds strong bones, especially in the elderly. Vitamin C is a very special water-soluble compound that helps the formation of bones, cartilage, muscle and blood vessels.

Cucumbers are available year round. You can eat the skin unless it has been treated with a protective coating of wax, in which case the skin should not be eaten.

Protein	2 g	Potassium	442 mg	Niacin (B3)	0.3 mg
Fat	0 g	Vitamin A	316 IU	Vitamin B6	0.1 mg
Carbohydrate	11 g	Vitamin C	8 mg	Folate	21 mcg
Calcium	48 mg	Vitamin D	~	Vitamin B12	0 mcg
Phosphorus	72 mg	Vitamin E	0.1 mg	Pantothenic Acid	0.8 mg
Magnesium	39 mg	Vitamin K	49 mcg	Dietary Fiber	1.5 g
Iron	0.8 mg	Thiamin (B1)	0.1 mg	Kilojoules (kJ)	189
Sodium	6 mg	Riboflavin (B2)	0.1 mg	Calories	45

EGGPLANT

Nutrients per 1 cup, cubed (82 g)

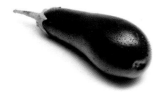

Excellent source of dietary fiber, potassium, copper, thiamin, riboflavin, niacin and pantothenic acid.

The most common variety of eggplant has a shiny, dark purple skin. Nasunin, an anthocyanin phytonutrient, is present in the skin of the eggplant. Nasunin is a powerful antioxidant and free-radical scavenger and may ward off damage to cell membranes. Eggplants are rich in certain compounds (phenolic) that function as antioxidants.

The high fiber content of the eggplant vegetable may act towards relieving occasional constipation, lowering the risk of hemorrhoids, which may help to protect the colon against certain cancers and diverticular disease.

Eggplant is available all year round and is at its most abundant from August to September. Brush with olive oil and grill thick slices.

Protein	1 g	Potassium	189 mg	Niacin (B3)	0.5 mg
Fat	0.2 g	Vitamin A	22 IU	Vitamin B6	0.1 mg
Carbohydrate	5 g	Vitamin C	2 mg	Folate	18 mcg
Calcium	7 mg	Vitamin D	~	Vitamin B12	0 mcg
Phosphorus	20 mg	Vitamin E	0.2 mg	Pantothenic Acid	0.2 mg
Magnesium	11 mg	Vitamin K	3 mcg	Dietary Fiber	3 g
Iron	0.2 mg	Thiamin (B1)	0 mg	Kilojoules (kJ)	82
Sodium	2 mg	Riboflavin (B2)	0 mg	Calories	19

GREEN BEANS

Nutrients per 1 cup (110 g)

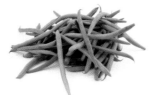

Excellent source of vitamin K, vitamin C and folate.
Good source of manganese, vitamin A and fiber.

Green beans are a favorite with those trying to lose weight because they are low in calories. The nutrients contained in green beans support healthy blood vessels and blood pressure and build strong bones. The iron in green beans assures a good energy supply and the fiber, vitamin C, folate and beta-carotene may be helpful in promoting colon health. All parts of the green bean may be eaten, although some people snip off the pointed ends because they can be stringy. Green beans are available in grocery stores year round.

Protein	2 g	Potassium	230 mg	Niacin (B3)	0.8 mg
Fat	0 g	Vitamin A	759 IU	Vitamin B6	0.1 mg
Carbohydrate	8 g	Vitamin C	18 mg	Folate	41 mcg
Calcium	41 mg	Vitamin D	~	Vitamin B12	0 mcg
Phosphorus	42 mg	Vitamin E	0.5 mg	Pantothenic Acid	0.1 mg
Magnesium	28 mg	Vitamin K	16 mcg	Dietary Fiber	4 g
Iron	1.1 mg	Thiamin (B1)	0.1 mg	Kilojoules (kJ)	143
Sodium	7 mg	Riboflavin (B2)	0.1 mg	Calories	34

KALE

Nutrients per 1 cup, chopped (67g)

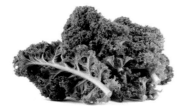

Excellent source of vitamins A, C and K and manganese.

Several studies have supported the claim that the nutrients in kale help heal eye-related damage and decrease risks of cataracts and macular degeneration.

The manganese in kale is a trace mineral and is useful in the production of energy from protein and carbohydrates. It may also supply a degree of protection against damage from free radicals produced during the production of energy.

There are several varieties of kale, and their color varies from green and white to purple and blue. Kale grows in cooler climates and tastes better after being exposed to frost. Available year round, kale is at its peak from mid-winter to early spring.

Protein	2 g	**Potassium**	299 mg	**Niacin (B3)**	0.7 mg
Fat	0 g	**Vitamin A**	10302 IU	**Vitamin B6**	0.2 mg
Carbohydrate	7 g	**Vitamin C**	80 mg	**Folate**	19 mcg
Calcium	90 mg	**Vitamin D**	~	**Vitamin B12**	0 mcg
Phosphorus	38 mg	**Vitamin E**	~	**Pantothenic Acid**	0.1 mg
Magnesium	23 mg	**Vitamin K**	547 mcg	**Dietary Fiber**	1 g
Iron	1.1 mg	**Thiamin (B1)**	0.1 mg	**Kilojoules (kJ)**	140
Sodium	29 mg	**Riboflavin (B2)**	0.1 mg	**Calories**	34

Regardless of which fruit and vegetables you purchase to juice, be sure to wash them well before juicing.

A glass of fresh juice helps to appease your appetite, so you don't want to eat as much.

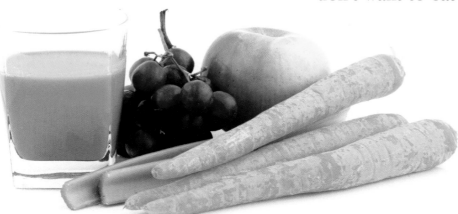

LEEKS

Nutrients per 1 cup (89 g)

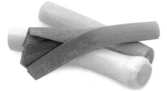

Excellent source of manganese, vitamin A and vitamin K.
Good source of iron, vitamin C and folate.

The leek's extended family consists of veggies such as onions, garlic, scallions and chives. The vegetables of this family have a strong reputation for helping prevent conditions such as high blood pressure and high cholesterol levels. When blood pressure and cholesterol levels are kept in check, this helps prevent heart attack and stroke. Research has indicated that this genus, known as the allium genus, may play a role in reducing the risk of developing certain cancers.

The white root end of the leek is edible. The darker green ends are very tough. This vegetable has a milder flavor than its cousins the onions and garlic. Leeks are available all year round and are at their peak in fall and winter. Make sure to slice into the leeks, soak them in cold water and wash them thoroughly before using. Using garden soil gets right inside, between the layers.

Protein	1 g	Potassium	160 mg	Niacin (B3)	0.4 mg
Fat	0 g	Vitamin A	1484 IU	Vitamin B6	0.2 mg
Carbohydrate	13 g	Vitamin C	11 mg	Folate	57 mcg
Calcium	53 mg	Vitamin D	~	Vitamin B12	0 mcg
Phosphorus	31 mg	Vitamin E	1 mg	Pantothenic Acid	0.1 mg
Magnesium	25 mg	Vitamin K	41 mcg	Dietary Fiber	2 g
Iron	1.9 mg	Thiamin (B1)	0.1 mg	Kilojoules (kJ)	227
Sodium	18 mg	Riboflavin (B2)	0 mg	Calories	54

ICEBERG LETTUCE

Nutrients per 1 cup, chopped (72g)

Good source of vitamin K.

On a diet? Iceberg lettuce may fit the bill perfectly. This vegetable may not be loaded with nutrition and others in the lettuce family might be a better choice, but it is packed with water and is extremely low in calories (only 10 in a cupful).

Iceberg lettuce does have a good amount of vitamin K, which is a fat-soluble vitamin that plays a role in blood clotting. It is also useful for the elderly, since vitamin K has a proven record of helping to maintain strong bones.

Iceberg lettuce is a very popular vegetable and is available year round, with its growing peak running from June to December.

Protein	0 g	Potassium	102 mg	Niacin (B3)	0.1 mg
Fat	0 g	Vitamin A	361 IU	Vitamin B6	0 mg
Carbohydrate	2 g	Vitamin C	2 mg	Folate	21 mcg
Calcium	13 mg	Vitamin D	~	Vitamin B12	0 mcg
Phosphorus	14 mg	Vitamin E	0.1 mg	Pantothenic Acid	0.1 mg
Magnesium	5 mg	Vitamin K	~	Dietary Fiber	1 g
Iron	1.3 mg	Thiamin (B1)	0 mg	Kilojoules (kJ)	24
Sodium	7 mg	Riboflavin (B2)	0 mg	Calories	10

ROMAINE LETTUCE

Nutrients per 1 cup, shredded (47g)

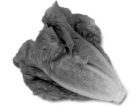

Excellent source of vitamins A and K.
Good source of vitamin C.

You can identify romaine lettuce by its elongated head and deep green outer leaves. Deep green is good. The deeper the color of our foods the better the nutrient value.

Vitamin K is a fat-soluble vitamin that greatly aids the role of blood clotting. The elderly can benefit significantly from vitamin K in that it is important in maintaining strong bones. Vitamin A is essential for the reproductive processes in both males and females in addition to helping normal bone metabolism.

Romaine lettuce is available year round.

Protein	1 g	Potassium	116 mg	Niacin (B3)	0.1 mg
Fat	0 g	Vitamin A	4094 IU	Vitamin B6	0 mg
Carbohydrate	2 g	Vitamin C	11 mg	Folate	64 mcg
Calcium	15 mg	Vitamin D	~	Vitamin B12	0 mcg
Phosphorus	14 mg	Vitamin E	0.1 mg	Pantothenic Acid	0.1 mg
Magnesium	7 mg	Vitamin K	48 mcg	Dietary Fiber	1 g
Iron	0.5 mg	Thiamin (B1)	0 mg	Kilojoules (kJ)	33
Sodium	4 mg	Riboflavin (B2)	0 mg	Calories	8

MUSHROOMS

Nutrients per 1 cup, sliced (70g)

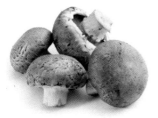

Good source of selenium.

Mushrooms are not a vegetable. They are a fungus. They contain no roots, leaves, seeds or flowers. Incredibly, there are an estimated 38,000 species of mushrooms, most of which supply protein, fiber, vitamins and other minerals. The selenium in mushrooms may help to reduce the risk of cardiovascular disease.

Also found in mushrooms is potassium, which helps maintain normal heart rhythm and fluid balance, muscle and nerve function.

Mushrooms in general are a fair source or riboflavin, niacin and pantothenic acid. Riboflavin helps promote good skin and vision. Niacin helps the digestive and nervous systems function properly and pantothenic acid aids in hormone production.

Mushrooms are generally available year round. Don't go eating wild mushrooms unless you are well trained to know which are poisonous and which are not.

Protein	2 g	Potassium	220 mg	Niacin (B3)	3 mg
Fat	0 g	Vitamin A	0 IU	Vitamin B6	0.1 mg
Carbohydrate	2 g	Vitamin C	2 mg	Folate	11 mcg
Calcium	2 mg	Vitamin D	~	Vitamin B12	0 mcg
Phosphorus	60 mg	Vitamin E	0 mg	Pantothenic Acid	1 mg
Magnesium	6 mg	Vitamin K	0 mcg	Dietary Fiber	1 g
Iron	0.3 mg	Thiamin (B1)	0.1 mg	Kilojoules (kJ)	65
Sodium	3 mg	Riboflavin (B2)	0.3 mg	Calories	15

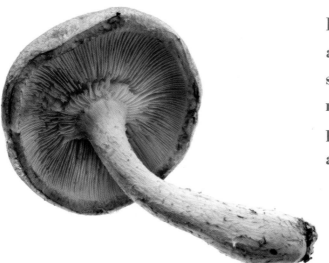

Incredibly, there are an estimated 38,000 species of mushrooms, most of which supply protein, fiber, vitamins and other minerals.

OKRA

Nutrients per 1 cup (100g)

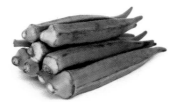

Excellent source of manganese, vitamin C, folate and vitamin A.
Good source of fiber, magnesium and thiamin.

South Americans used okra seeds as a coffee substitute during the Civil War, and these seeds are still used as a fine substitute for coffee. Okra is a green vegetable that packs a lot of punch. Okra contains both vitamin C and manganese, nutrients the physique athlete requires to build up joints and cartilage. Vitamin C's role as an antioxidant is linked to a reduced risk of heart disease. The nervous system and brain have many uses for folate, including preventing dementia. Magnesium is of prime importance to seniors in that it contributes to good heart health. The best okra is available between September and October.

Protein	2 g	Potassium	303 mg	Niacin (B3)	1 mg
Fat	0.1 g	Vitamin A	375 IU	Vitamin B6	0.2 mg
Carbohydrate	7 g	Vitamin C	21 mg	Folate	88 mcg
Calcium	81 mg	Vitamin D	~	Vitamin B12	0 mcg
Phosphorus	63 mg	Vitamin E	0.4 mg	Pantothenic Acid	0.2 mg
Magnesium	57 mg	Vitamin K	53 mcg	Dietary Fiber	3 g
Iron	0.8 mg	Thiamin (B1)	0.2 mg	Kilojoules (kJ)	130
Sodium	8 mg	Riboflavin (B2)	0.1 mg	Calories	31

ONIONS

Nutrients per 1 cup, chopped (160 g)

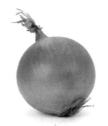

Good source of vitamin C and manganese.

Onions are rich in chromium, a trace mineral that helps you maintain normal blood-sugar levels. Onions may also help with maladies such as arthritis and the allergic inflammation of asthma. The combination of quercetin and other flavonoids found in onions along with vitamin C may help inhibit bacteria.

Onion varieties include yellow onions, white onions (which have a high water content), Spanish onions, and red onions (from Bermuda). Scallions are long and slender. Shallots are firm, violet-tinged bulbs.

Many onions are available year round.

Protein	2 g	Potassium	234 mg	Niacin (B3)	0.2 mg
Fat	0 g	Vitamin A	3 IU	Vitamin B6	0.2 mg
Carbohydrate	15 g	Vitamin C	12 mg	Folate	30 mcg
Calcium	37 mg	Vitamin D	~	Vitamin B12	0 mcg
Phosphorus	46 mg	Vitamin E	0 mg	Pantothenic Acid	0.2 mg
Magnesium	16 mg	Vitamin K	1 mcg	Dietary Fiber	3 g
Iron	0.3 mg	Thiamin (B1)	0.1 mg	Kilojoules (kJ)	268
Sodium	6 mg	Riboflavin (B2)	0 mg	Calories	64

PARSNIPS

Nutrients per 1 cup, sliced (133 g)

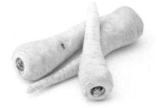

Excellent source of fiber, manganese, vitamin C, folate and vitamin K.
Good source of potassium.

Parsnips are an excellent source of the water-soluble antioxidant vitamin C. They are low in fat, cholesterol and sodium.

Vitamin C may help protect against inflammation, which may play a role in heart disease, certain cancers and asthma. Folic acid, too, may play a part in reducing the risk of heart disease and stroke.

Fiber plays an important part in relieving occasional constipation, which may help to reduce hemorrhoids and other complications of the bowel. It also plays an important role in weight control.

Vitamin K is vital for blood clotting and maintaining strong bones.

Parsnips are available year round, with peak season being April to October.

Protein	2 g	Potassium	499 mg	Niacin (B3)	0.9 mg
Fat	0 g	Vitamin A	0 IU	Vitamin B6	0.1 mg
Carbohydrate	24 g	Vitamin C	23 mg	Folate	89 mcg
Calcium	48 mg	Vitamin D	~	Vitamin B12	0 mcg
Phosphorus	94 mg	Vitamin E	2 mg	Pantothenic Acid	1 mg
Magnesium	39 mg	Vitamin K	29.9 mcg	Dietary Fiber	6 g
Iron	0.8 mg	Thiamin (B1)	0.1 mg	Kilojoules (kJ)	418
Sodium	13 mg	Riboflavin (B2)	0.1 mg	Calories	100

PEAS, GREEN

Nutrients per 1 cup (145 g)

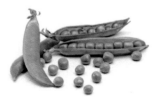

Excellent source of vitamins K, C and A. Good source of protein, fiber, iron, magnesium, potassium, manganese, thiamin, pantothenic acid and folate.

Green peas are an excellent source of vitamin K, which works to keep calcium inside the bone. Vitamin K is also needed for blood clotting. The high vitamin C content in green peas helps the adrenal glands, ocular lens, liver, immune system and connective tissues. Amazingly, there are more than 1,000 varieties of peas. Most popular varieties are sugar snap peas and snow peas, both of which have edible pods. Dried peas are usually available year round. Peas are a lentil and have the lentil's proclivity to contain protein.

Protein	8 g	Potassium	354 mg	Niacin (B3)	3 mg
Fat	1 g	Vitamin A	1109 IU	Vitamin B6	0.2 mg
Carbohydrate	21 g	Vitamin C	58 mg	Folate	94 mcg
Calcium	36 mg	Vitamin D	~	Vitamin B12	0 mcg
Phosphorus	157 mg	Vitamin E	0.2 mg	Pantothenic Acid	0.2 mg
Magnesium	48 mg	Vitamin K	36 mcg	Dietary Fiber	7 g
Iron	2.1 mg	Thiamin (B1)	0.4 mg	Kilojoules (kJ)	490
Sodium	7 mg	Riboflavin (B2)	0.2 mg	Calories	117

PEPPERS, BELL

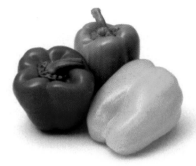

Excellent source of vitamin C.
Good source of vitamin K (beta-carotene).

Healthy cholesterol is in part the result of the combination of vitamin C and beta-carotene working together, and this pairing also helps nerve and blood vessels, eyesight and lung function.

Bell peppers, known also as sweet peppers, come in a variety of colors: green, red, yellow, orange, purple, black and brown. Red peppers contain lycopene (which may help reduce the risk of prostate cancer). Inside the pepper is an inner cavity that contains edible seeds and a white spongy core. The green variety has a slightly bitter flavor, but the red, orange and yellows are sweeter.

Peppers are available year round, with their peak season from July through September.

RED

Nutrients per 1 medium
red bell pepper (119 g)

Protein	1 g	**Potassium**	251 mg	**Niacin (B3)**	1.2 mg
Fat	0 g	**Vitamin A**	3726 IU	**Vitamin B6**	0.3 mg
Carbohydrate	7 g	**Vitamin C**	152 mg	**Folate**	55 mcg
Calcium	8 mg	**Vitamin D**	~	**Vitamin B12**	0 mcg
Phosphorus	31 mg	**Vitamin E**	2 mg	**Pantothenic Acid**	0.4 mg
Magnesium	14 mg	**Vitamin K**	6 mcg	**Dietary Fiber**	3 g
Iron	0.5 mg	**Thiamin (B1)**	0.1 mg	**Kilojoules (kJ)**	154
Sodium	5 mg	**Riboflavin (B2)**	0.1 mg	**Calories**	37

GREEN

Nutrients per 1 medium
green bell pepper (119 g)

Protein	1 g	**Potassium**	208 mg	**Niacin (B3)**	0.6 mg
Fat	0 g	**Vitamin A**	440 IU	**Vitamin B6**	0.3 mg
Carbohydrate	6 g	**Vitamin C**	96 mg	**Folate**	12 mcg
Calcium	12 mg	**Vitamin D**	~	**Vitamin B12**	0 mcg
Phosphorus	24 mg	**Vitamin E**	0.4 mg	**Pantothenic Acid**	0.1 mg
Magnesium	12 mg	**Vitamin K**	9 mcg	**Dietary Fiber**	2 g
Iron	0.4 mg	**Thiamin (B1)**	0.1 mg	**Kilojoules (kJ)**	100
Sodium	4 mg	**Riboflavin (B2)**	0 mg	**Calories**	24

POTATOES

Nutrients per 1 medium potato (213 g)

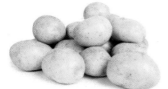

Excellent source of vitamin B6, potassium and vitamin C. Good source of fiber, iron, magnesium, phosphorus, copper, manganese, niacin (vitamin B3) and folate.

The formatting of new cells is aided by vitamin B6, which helps break down the sugar stored in muscle cells and in the liver, making it important in both endurance and athletic performance. Vitamin B6 may also help to reduce the risk of cancer and heart disease.

The fiber is contained mainly in the potato skin, so if you want the fiber you will have to eat the skin. There are about 100 varieties of potatoes.

Large potatoes generally are referred to as "mature" while the smaller varieties are called "new." The skin of the potato can be brown, red or yellow. Potatoes store well and are available throughout the year.

Protein	4 g	Potassium	897 mg	Niacin (B3)	2.2 mg
Fat	0 g	Vitamin A	4 IU	Vitamin B6	0.6 mg
Carbohydrate	39 g	Vitamin C	42 mg	Folate	34 mcg
Calcium	26 mg	Vitamin D	~	Vitamin B12	0 mcg
Phosphorus	121 mg	Vitamin E	0 mg	Pantothenic Acid	0.6 mg
Magnesium	49 mg	Vitamin K	4 mcg	Dietary Fiber	5 g
Iron	1.7 mg	Thiamin (B1)	0.1 mg	Kilojoules (kJ)	687
Sodium	13 mg	Riboflavin (B2)	0.1 mg	Calories	164

PUMPKIN

Nutrients per 1 cup, cubed (116g)

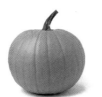

Excellent source of vitamin A. Good source of potassium and vitamin C.

The pumpkin contains beta-carotene and alpha-carotene, which convert to vitamin A, a fat-soluble vitamin responsible for healthy skin, hair and mucous membranes. It may help support healthy eyesight and may be important for tooth development, bone growth and reproduction. Pumpkins are a good source of vitamin C and a powerful antioxidant and anti-inflammatory.

Pumpkin seeds (roasted) make a tasty snack and offer significant protection to the prostate.

Fresh pumpkins are available from October through winter.

Protein	1 g	Potassium	394 mg	Niacin (B3)	0.7 mg
Fat	0 g	Vitamin A	8567 IU	Vitamin B6	0.1 mg
Carbohydrate	7 g	Vitamin C	10 mg	Folate	19 mcg
Calcium	24 mg	Vitamin D	~	Vitamin B12	0 mcg
Phosphorus	51 mg	Vitamin E	1 mg	Pantothenic Acid	0.3 mg
Magnesium	14 mg	Vitamin K	1 mcg	Dietary Fiber	1 g
Iron	0.9 mg	Thiamin (B1)	0.1 mg	Kilojoules (kJ)	129
Sodium	1 mg	Riboflavin (B2)	0.1 mg	Calories	30

RADICCHIO

Nutrients per 2 1/2 cups, raw (100 g)

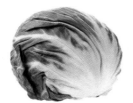

Good source of vitamin C, copper and folate.

Radicchio is a round, lettuce-like vegetable with dark burgundy leaves and contrasting white veins. It resembles a small cabbage. The leaves are easy to peel and offer a distinct bittersweet flavor.

Vitamin C, a powerful antioxidant, helps to build and maintain skin, bones, teeth, eyes, muscle, blood vessels and cartilage. The immune system benefits greatly from this vitamin.

Folate is required for the building of energy and the formation of blood cells. It is important for pregnant women to increase their intake of folic acid to help reduce the risk of birth defects, and is thought to help prevent heart disease, Parkinson's and Alzheimer's.

Protein	1 g	Potassium	302 mg	Niacin (B3)	0.2 mg
Fat	0 g	Vitamin A	27 IU	Vitamin B6	0 mg
Carbohydrate	4 g	Vitamin C	8 mg	Folate	60 mcg
Calcium	18 mg	Vitamin D	~	Vitamin B12	0 mcg
Phosphorus	40 mg	Vitamin E	2 mg	Pantothenic Acid	0.2 mg
Magnesium	13 mg	Vitamin K	255 mcg	Dietary Fiber	1 g
Iron	0.5 mg	Thiamin (B1)	0 mg	Kilojoules (kJ)	95
Sodium	22 mg	Riboflavin (B2)	0 mg	Calories	23

RADISHES

Nutrients per 1 cup (116g)

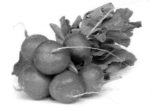

Excellent source of vitamin C.

Radishes are an excellent source of vitamin C and are virtually fat free and very low in calories. They are an ideal food for anyone preparing for a physique contest or modeling assignment – or simply a beach vacation – where the body is on show. Radishes are also cholesterol free and very low in sodium. Vitamin C is an antioxidant that is recognized as one of the most important vitamins.

Decreasing fat in the diet can help improve health and reduce the risk of certain cancers. And the decrease in sodium may reduce the risk of hypertension.

Radishes are available year round, but are best in early winter.

Protein	1 g	Potassium	270 mg	Niacin (B3)	0.3 mg
Fat	0.1 g	Vitamin A	8 IU	Vitamin B6	0.1 mg
Carbohydrate	4 g	Vitamin C	17 mg	Folate	29 mcg
Calcium	29 mg	Vitamin D	~	Vitamin B12	0 mcg
Phosphorus	23 mg	Vitamin E	0 mg	Pantothenic Acid	0.2 mg
Magnesium	12 mg	Vitamin K	2 mcg	Dietary Fiber	2 g
Iron	0.4 mg	Thiamin (B1)	0 mg	Kilojoules (kJ)	77
Sodium	45 mg	Riboflavin (B2)	0 mg	Calories	19

SOYBEANS

Nutrients per 1 cup (256 g)

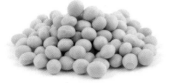

Excellent source of protein, fiber, calcium, iron, magnesium, phosphorus, potassium, manganese, vitamin C, thiamin and folate.
Good source of zinc, copper, riboflavin and niacin.

The seeds of the soybean, which grow in pods, are edible. Soybeans are an excellent source of protein. Scientists have noted that soy protein lowers blood cholesterol levels while animal protein tends to raise blood cholesterol levels. Soy protein also helps to lower blood pressure, thus protecting against heart disease and stroke. Soybeans may also support kidney function because they are easier on the kidneys than animal protein.

The high fiber content may also help reduce the risk of certain cancers. It may also reduce the symptoms of irritable bowel syndrome. Soybeans and soy foods are available year round.

Protein	33 g	**Potassium**	1587 mg	**Niacin (B3)**	4.2 mg
Fat	17 g	**Vitamin A**	461 IU	**Vitamin B6**	0.2 mg
Carbohydrate	28 g	**Vitamin C**	74 mg	**Folate**	422 mcg
Calcium	504 mg	**Vitamin D**	~	**Vitamin B12**	0 mcg
Phosphorus	497 mg	**Vitamin E**	0 mg	**Pantothenic Acid**	0.4 mg
Magnesium	166 mg	**Vitamin K**	0 mcg	**Dietary Fiber**	11 g
Iron	9.1 mg	**Thiamin (B1)**	1.1 mg	**Kilojoules (kJ)**	1574
Sodium	38 mg	**Riboflavin (B2)**	0.4 mg	**Calories**	376

The seeds of the soybean, called edamame, are edible. These are usually found in the frozen vegetable section.

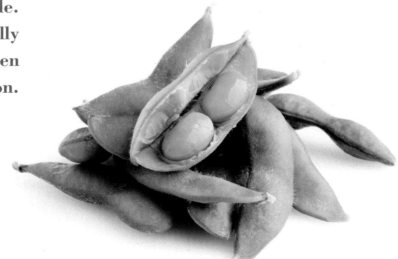

SPINACH

Nutrients per 1 cup (30g)

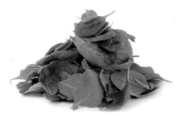

Excellent source of vitamin A and vitamin K.
Good source of manganese, vitamin C and folate.

Spinach is a highly nutritious food that every kitchen should contain. Osteo-calcin is activated by the abundance of vitamin K in spinach, and consequently helps to maintain healthy bones. Osteocalcin anchors calcium molecules inside the bone. Vitamin K is also needed for blood clotting. The C and A vitamins are important antioxidants.

Folate is found in spinach and is important for reducing the risk of heart attacks and stroke. Foods high in vitamin C, beta-carotene and folate may lower the risk of certain cancers.

There are three varieties of spinach, savoy, semi-savoy and smooth leaf. Spinach is available year round but it is at its best in fall and spring.

Protein	1 g	Potassium	167 mg	Niacin (B3)	0.2 mg
Fat	0.1 g	Vitamin A	2813 IU	Vitamin B6	0.1 mg
Carbohydrate	1 g	Vitamin C	8 mg	Folate	58 mcg
Calcium	30 mg	Vitamin D	~	Vitamin B12	0 mcg
Phosphorus	15 mg	Vitamin E	0.6 mg	Pantothenic Acid	0 mg
Magnesium	24 mg	Vitamin K	145 mcg	Dietary Fiber	1 g
Iron	0.8 mg	Thiamin (B1)	0 mg	Kilojoules (kJ)	29
Sodium	24 mg	Riboflavin (B2)	0.1 mg	Calories	7

SQUASH

Nutrients per 1 cup, cubed, (140 g)

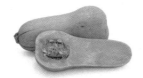

Excellent source of vitamin C and Vitamin A. Good source of vitamin B6.

The vitamin C and beta-carotene in squash may help to keep cholesterol levels under control. Vitamin B6 and folate are required to maintain healthy homo-cystein levels. In fact, high homocystein levels are associated with risk of heart attack and stroke, so regulation is important.

Folate, vitamin C and beta-carotene may help prevent colon cancer. They may also have anti-inflammatory properties that could benefit arthritis and asthma. All of squash is edible and varieties include zucchini, crookneck and straight neck.

Protein	1 g	Potassium	493 mg	Niacin (B3)	1.7 mg
Fat	0 g	Vitamin A	14883 IU	Vitamin B6	0.2 mg
Carbohydrate	16 g	Vitamin C	29 mg	Folate	38 mcg
Calcium	67 mg	Vitamin D	~	Vitamin B12	0 mcg
Phosphorus	46 mg	Vitamin E	2 mg	Pantothenic Acid	0.6 mg
Magnesium	47 mg	Vitamin K	2 mcg	Dietary Fiber	3 g
Iron	1 mg	Thiamin (B1)	0.1 mg	Kilojoules (kJ)	264
Sodium	6 mg	Riboflavin (B2)	0 mg	Calories	63

SWEET POTATO

Nutrients per 1 whole,
5 inches long (130 g)

Excellent source of vitamins A, C, and B6, manganese, fiber and potassium.
Good source of magnesium, phosphorus, copper, thiamin, riboflavin, niacin, and
pantothenic acid.

The sweet potato is a starchy carbohydrate that has become a great favorite among fitness athletes for its high nutritional value, lovely sweet flavor and low glycemic index.

Vitamin C and vitamin A (beta-carotene) are antioxidants, which research has indicated may reduce the risk of heart disease, stroke and certain cancers.

Vitamin B6 helps reduce homocystein levels. High homocystein levels may be linked to increased risk of heart attacks or strokes. Although future research is needed, the proteins in sweet potatoes appear to have strong anti-oxidant capabilities.

Different types of sweet potatoes abound. They can be found in a variety of colors including white, yellow, orange, red or purple. They store well and are readily available year round.

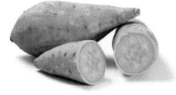

Protein	2 g	**Potassium**	438 mg	**Niacin (B3)**	0.7 mg
Fat	0 g	**Vitamin A**	18441 IU	**Vitamin B6**	0.3 mg
Carbohydrate	26 g	**Vitamin C**	3 mg	**Folate**	14 mcg
Calcium	39 mg	**Vitamin D**	~	**Vitamin B12**	0 mcg
Phosphorus	61 mg	**Vitamin E** (Alpha Tocopherol)	0.3 mg	**Pantothenic Acid**	1 mg
Magnesium	33 mg	**Vitamin K**	2 mcg	**Dietary Fiber**	4 g
Iron	0.8 mg	**Thiamin (B1)**	0.1 mg	**Kilojoules (kJ)**	469
Sodium	71 mg	**Riboflavin (B2)**	0.1 mg	**Calories**	112

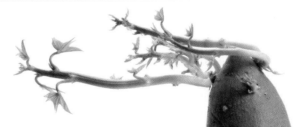

The sweet potato has become a great favorite among fitness athletes for its high nutritional value, lovely sweet flavor and low glycemic index.

SWISS CHARD

Nutrients per 1 cup (36 g)

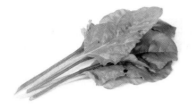

Excellent source of vitamin K, vitamin A, magnesium, vitamin C, potassium, iron and manganese. Good source of fiber, copper and calcium.

Chard is a fall leafy vegetable. Vitamin K is needed for bone health and is necessary to create osteocalcin, which is a non-collagen protein in bone.

Vitamin A and beta-carotene are essential to support good vision. Magnesium may help control high blood pressure, spasms of the muscular system including the heart muscle, and the network of airways. Deficiency of magnesium has been associated with severe headaches (migraine), muscle cramps, soreness and fatigue. Vitamin C may help promote a healthy cardiovascular system.

Correct blood pressure and heart function is helped with potassium. The iron content in Swiss chard enhances oxygen distribution throughout the body. Fiber helps maintain healthy blood sugar levels and may help reduce colon cancer.

Chard is available year round but is most abundant from June to August.

Protein	1 g	Potassium	136 mg	Niacin (B3)	0.1 mg
Fat	0 g	Vitamin A	2202 IU	Vitamin B6	0 mg
Carbohydrate	1 g	Vitamin C	11 mg	Folate	5 mcg
Calcium	18 mg	Vitamin D	~	Vitamin B12	0 mcg
Phosphorus	17 mg	Vitamin E	1 mg	Pantothenic Acid	0.1 mg
Magnesium	29 mg	Vitamin K	299 mcg	Dietary Fiber	1 g
Iron	0.6 mg	Thiamin (B1)	0 mg	Kilojoules (kJ)	29
Sodium	77 mg	Riboflavin (B2)	0 mg	Calories	7

A glass of fresh juice keeps your energy level up while making your taste buds dance with delight.

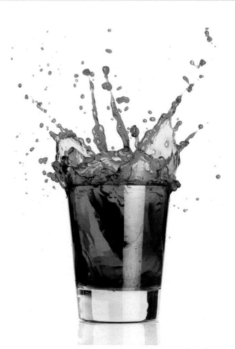

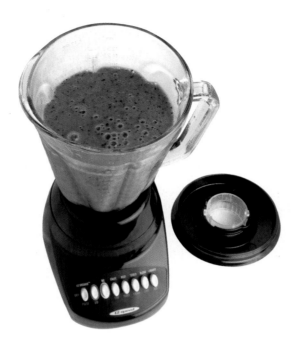

Juicing is a wonderful way to get nature's freshness into your body.

TOMATOES

Nutrients per 1 medium tomato (123 g)

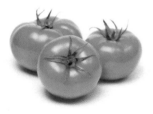

Excellent source of vitamin C and vitamin A. Good source of vitamin K.

Tomatoes are one of the most popular vegetables, but are in fact a fruit. They were at one time thought to be poisonous until a market merchant in Spain started eating them in public in order to sell them to the Spanish citizens.

Research has shown that the eating of tomatoes may be beneficial against the risk of developing prostate cancer (the lycopene that helps prevent prostate cancer is more bioavailable with cooked tomato), colon cancer, rectal cancer and cervical cancer.

Tomatoes come in a large variety of colors, sizes and shapes, including heirloom tomatoes (which taste wonderful), yellow or orange tomatoes, cherry tomatoes, roma, grape and pear tomatoes.

They are grown in every state and province of North America and are available year round.

Protein	1 g	**Potassium**	292 mg	**Niacin (B3)**	0.7 mg
Fat	0.2 g	**Vitamin A**	1025 IU	**Vitamin B6**	0.1 mg
Carbohydrate	5 g	**Vitamin C**	16 mg	**Folate**	18 mcg
Calcium	12 mg	**Vitamin D**	~	**Vitamin B12**	0 mcg
Phosphorus	29 mg	**Vitamin E**	0.7 mg	**Pantothenic Acid**	0.1 mg
Magnesium	13 mg	**Vitamin K**	10 mcg	**Dietary Fiber**	2 g
Iron	0.3 mg	**Thiamin (B1)**	0 mg	**Kilojoules (kJ)**	92
Sodium	6 mg	**Riboflavin (B2)**	0 mg	**Calories**	22

TURNIPS

Nutrients per 1 cup, cubed (130 g)

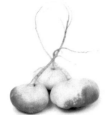

Excellent source of vitamin C. Good source of fiber, potassium and manganese.

Turnips are usually a light beige in color, with an occasional appearance of purple. They are a root vegetable, grown underground. Small turnips tend to be sweeter than the larger varieties. They can be eaten raw or cooked. The high vitamin C content in turnips makes them a powerful antioxidant. Vitamin C gives foundation to cartilage, bones, muscle and blood vessels, helping the body to heal wounds and resist infection.

Early studies of vitamin C indicate that some effects associated with asthma may be helped by its inclusion in the diet. Turnips store well and are available year round.

Protein	1 g	Potassium	248 mg	Niacin (B3)	0.5 mg
Fat	0.1 g	Vitamin A	0 IU	Vitamin B6	0.1 mg
Carbohydrate	8 g	Vitamin C	27 mg	Folate	20 mcg
Calcium	39 mg	Vitamin D	~	Vitamin B12	0 mcg
Phosphorus	35 mg	Vitamin E	0 mg	Pantothenic Acid	0.3 mg
Magnesium	14 mg	Vitamin K	0.1 mcg	Dietary Fiber	2 g
Iron	0.4 mg	Thiamin (B1)	0 mg	Kilojoules (kJ)	152
Sodium	87 mg	Riboflavin (B2)	0 mg	Calories	36

WATERCRESS

Nutrients per 1 cup, chopped (34 g)

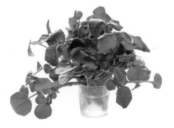

Excellent source of vitamins A and K.
Good source of vitamin C.

The antioxidants in watercress may help reduce the risk of developing certain cancers. Studies are currently underway to confirm this. There is evidence that they may also support healthy cholesterol levels.

Watercress is an excellent source of vitamin A (beta-carotene), which helps humans develop and maintain healthy skin and eyes and contributes strongly to healthy vision. Vitamin K helps maintain strong bones and helps blood clotting. This is especially important for the elderly.

Watercress is available in most grocery stores year round.

Protein	1 g	Potassium	112 mg	Niacin (B3)	0.1 mg
Fat	0 g	Vitamin A	1058 IU	Vitamin B6	0 mg
Carbohydrate	0 g	Vitamin C	15 mg	Folate	3 mcg
Calcium	41 mg	Vitamin D	~	Vitamin B12	0 mcg
Phosphorus	20 mg	Vitamin E	0.3 mg	Pantothenic Acid	0.1 mg
Magnesium	7 mg	Vitamin K	85 mcg	Dietary Fiber	0.2 g
Iron	0.1 mg	Thiamin (B1)	0 mg	Kilojoules (kJ)	16
Sodium	14 mg	Riboflavin (B2)	0 mg	Calories	4

YAMS

Nutrients per 1 cup, cubed (150 g)

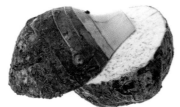

Excellent source of fiber, potassium, vitamin C and vitamin B6.
Good source of copper and thiamin.

The yam is a bulb (a tube) of a tropical vine. They are not easily found in grocery stores in the U.S. or Canada. You may have to go to a grocery store that specializes in tropical foods in order to find them. What we call yams are most often actually sweet potatoes. Amazingly, a true yam can grow as large as 5 feet and weigh 120 pounds!

Yams contain a substantial amount of vitamin C, a water-soluble vitamin that may help prevent certain cancers.

Yams are also an excellent source of fiber, which may reduce the risk of colon abnormalities including cancer.

The natural coloring beta-carotene is found in yams. Beta-carotene converts in the body to vitamin A.

Warning: Yams must be cooked. They can be toxic if eaten raw.

Protein	2 g	Potassium	1224 mg	Niacin (B3)	0.8 mg
Fat	0.3 g	Vitamin A	207 IU	Vitamin B6	0.4 mg
Carbohydrate	42 g	Vitamin C	26 mg	Folate	35 mcg
Calcium	26 mg	Vitamin D	~	Vitamin B12	0 mcg
Phosphorus	82 mg	Vitamin E	0.5 mg	Pantothenic Acid	0.5 mg
Magnesium	32 mg	Vitamin K	3 mcg	Dietary Fiber	6 g
Iron	0.8 mg	Thiamin (B1)	0.2 mg	Kilojoules (kJ)	741
Sodium	14 mg	Riboflavin (B2)	0 mg	Calories	177

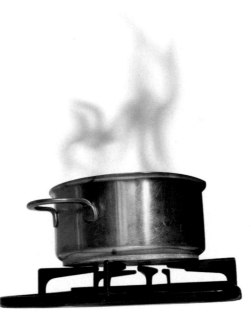

Yams must be cooked. They can be toxic if eaten raw.

GRAINS

From the beginning of civilization grains have been honored as healthy foods. Like most fruits and vegetables they help provide the body with essential vitamins and minerals, phytochemicals, protein and antioxidants.

While some of these nutritional values may sound just like what you get from vegetables and fruit, it's important to add grains to your diet because grains contain some nutrients that are not found in fruits and vegetables. The American Heart Association recommends we eat three servings of whole grains daily in addition to raw fruits and vegetables. There is currently no recommended daily allowance established for grains, but preliminary studies have shown that three or more servings of whole grains may help to reduce the risk of heart disease, stroke, cancer and diabetes.

BARLEY

Nutrients per 1 cup raw (200 g)

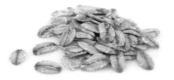

Excellent source of protein, fiber, iron, magnesium, phosphorus, potassium, zinc, copper, manganese, selenium, thiamin, riboflavin, niacin and vitamin B6.

Barley is a cereal grain rich in healthy nutrients. It is great for overall intestinal health and well-being.

The fiber in barley provides food for the friendly bacteria in the large intestine and is a great aid towards maintaining a healthy colon. Lower cholesterol levels may also become a reality as a result of the ingested dietary fiber.

Niacin is a B vitamin that may support cardiovascular health and reduce cholesterol levels.

Barley is available year round in many forms: pearl barley, scotch barley, hulled barley, barley flakes and barley grits.

Protein	20 g	Potassium	560 mg	Niacin (B3)	9.2 mg
Fat	2 g	Vitamin A	44 IU	Vitamin B6	0.5 mg
Carbohydrate	155 g	Vitamin C	0 mg	Folate	46 mcg
Calcium	58 mg	Vitamin D	~	Vitamin B12	0 mcg
Phosphorus	442 mg	Vitamin E	0 mg	Pantothenic Acid	0.6 mg
Magnesium	158 mg	Vitamin K	4 mcg	Dietary Fiber	31 g
Iron	5 mg	Thiamin (B1)	0.4 mg	Kilojoules (kJ)	2948
Sodium	18 mg	Riboflavin (B2)	0.2 mg	Calories	614

BRAN

Nutrients per 1 cup (94 g)

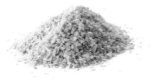

Excellent source of protein, fiber, iron, magnesium, phosphorus, zinc, copper, manganese, selenium, thiamin, niacin and vitamin B6.

The outer husk of wheat, rice, oats and other cereals is called bran. Each type of bran has its own properties. Wheat bran is mostly insoluble, absorbs large amounts of water and may help keep bowels regular. Oat bran is loaded with soluble fiber and among other things helps to regulate blood sugar. Rice bran reduces cholesterol levels. It is important to know that diets high in bran and other high-fiber foods can help play a role in weight control, thus reducing the risk of obesity.

Many whole-grain breads and cereals contain bran.

Protein	16 g	Potassium	532 mg	Niacin (B3)	0.9 mg
Fat	7 g	Vitamin A	0 IU	Vitamin B6	0.2 mg
Carbohydrate	62 g	Vitamin C	0 mg	Folate	49 mcg
Calcium	54 mg	Vitamin D	~	Vitamin B12	0 mcg
Phosphorus	690 mg	Vitamin E	1 mg	Pantothenic Acid	1.4 mg
Magnesium	221 mg	Vitamin K	3 mcg	Dietary Fiber	14 g
Iron	5.1 mg	Thiamin (B1)	1.1 mg	Kilojoules (kJ)	967
Sodium	4 mg	Riboflavin (B2)	0.2 mg	Calories	231

BROWN RICE

Nutrients per 1 cup dry (190 g)

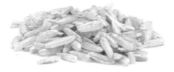

Excellent source of potassium and fiber. Good source of vitamin B3 and selenium.

Brown rice is eaten all over the world and is considered a very important food, especially in countries with many underprivileged people. When only the outermost layer of the rice bulb is removed we have brown rice. When further milling is involved, the brown rice becomes white rice. White rice is more popular and common; however, nutrients are lost in the milling process.

Brown rice may help keep the colon healthy and help prevent diseases of the colon. Selenium may decrease the symptoms of asthma and rheumatoid arthritis. Fiber helps to support healthy blood sugar and cholesterol levels.

Brown rice is available in most grocery stores.

Protein	14 g	Potassium	509 mg	Niacin (B3)	8.2 mg
Fat	5 g	Vitamin A	0 IU	Vitamin B6	1 mg
Carbohydrate	145 g	Vitamin C	0 mg	Folate	38 mcg
Calcium	63 mg	Vitamin D	~	Vitamin B12	0 mcg
Phosphorus	502 mg	Vitamin E	~	Pantothenic Acid	3 mg
Magnesium	272 mg	Vitamin K	~	Dietary Fiber	7 g
Iron	2.7 mg	Thiamin (B1)	0.8 mg	Kilojoules (kJ)	2881
Sodium	8 mg	Riboflavin (B2)	0.1 mg	Calories	688

OATS

Nutrients per 1 cup dry (156 g)

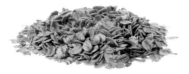

Excellent source of potassium and fiber. Good source of vitamin B1.

Oats, oat bran and oatmeal all contain beta-glucan fiber, which may play a role in controlling cholesterol levels.

Because of its amazing nutritional profile, hot oatmeal with berries has proven a favorite with experienced fitness enthusiasts as their first meal of the day (often followed by scrambled egg whites).

Oats may be beneficial in helping prevent heart disease, stroke and blood clots. There is an additional benefit in that oats have been found to stabilize blood sugars in non-insulin dependant diabetic patients.

Incidents of colon cancer are reduced in those who regularly consume oats.

Protein	26 g	Potassium	669 mg	Niacin (B3)	1.5 mg
Fat	11 g	Vitamin A	0 IU	Vitamin B6	0.2 mg
Carbohydrate	103 g	Vitamin C	0 mg	Folate	87 mcg
Calcium	84 mg	Vitamin D	~	Vitamin B12	0 mcg
Phosphorus	816 mg	Vitamin E)	~	Pantothenic Acid	2.1 mg
Magnesium	276 mg	Vitamin K	~	Dietary Fiber	16 g
Iron	7.4 mg	Thiamin (B1)	1.2 mg	Kilojoules (kJ)	2541
Sodium	3 mg	Riboflavin (B2)	0.2 mg	Calories	607

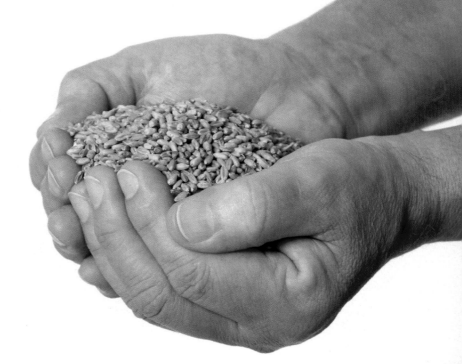

Try eating wheat in it's completely unrefined state, as wheat berries.

WHEAT

Nutrients per 1-cup
whole-grain flour (120 g)

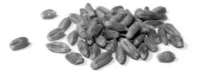

Excellent source of protein, fiber, iron, magnesium, phosphorus, zinc, copper, manganese, selenium, thiamin, niacin and vitamin B6.

Good source of potassium, riboflavin, pantothenic acid and folate.

Wheat is a grain grown worldwide. It is used in bread, pitas, bagels, wraps, noodles, crackers and cakes. The closer to its most natural state the better it is for you (not crackers or sugar-loaded refined cereals).

Wheat bran acts as a laxative, which may relieve some symptoms of diverticular disease. Wheat germ is a separate ingredient, removed from the whole wheat when the grain is refined. It is high in vitamin E and is important in the maintenance of a healthy immune system. Try eating wheat in its completely unrefined state, as wheat berries — chewy and delicious in salads and pilafs.

Caution: Individuals with untreated gallbladder or kidney problems may want to avoid whole wheat. See your doctor.

Protein	16 g	**Potassium**	486 mg	**Niacin (B3)**	7.6 mg
Fat	2 g	**Vitamin A**	11 IU	**Vitamin B6**	0.4 mg
Carbohydrate	87 g	**Vitamin C**	0 mg	**Folate**	53 mcg
Calcium	41 mg	**Vitamin D**	~	**Vitamin B12**	0 mcg
Phosphorus	415 mg	**Vitamin E**	1 mg	**Pantothenic Acid**	1.2 mg
Magnesium	166 mg	**Vitamin K**	2 mcg	**Dietary Fiber**	15 g
Iron	4.7 mg	**Thiamin (B1)**	0.5 mg	**Kilojoules (kJ)**	1702
Sodium	6 mg	**Riboflavin (B2)**	0.3 mg	**Calories**	407

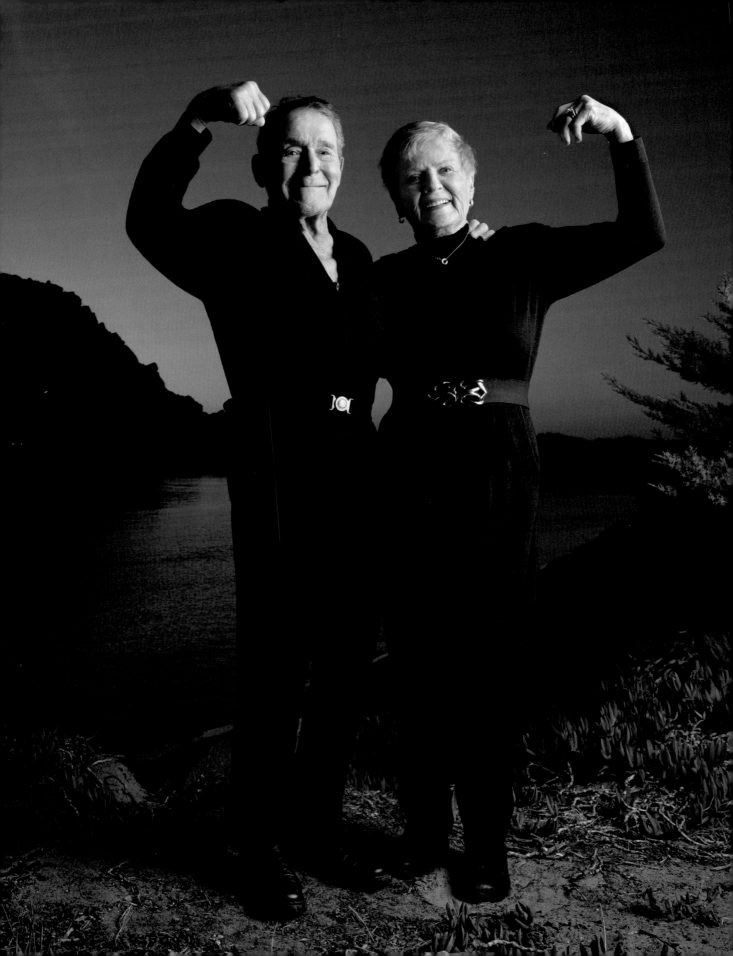

CHAPTER SIXTEEN

My Wish For You

Early on in this book I asked you to allow me to take you by the hand and lead you to a new and exciting lifestyle. I also admitted that I have no idea whether you are a man or woman, fat or thin, young or not so young. Nor does it matter.

What is high on my list is the burning desire to help you improve your life. As a teenager my own life was in the dumps and rapidly getting worse. I was angry with the world and I could have ended up in trouble. But as luck would have it, my life improved when I was inspired by a lecture on nutrition by Paul Bragg and by joining the Berkeley YMCA. There I learned to wrestle, and that's where I discovered weights. In fact, in those early years, I was so inspired I bought *Gray's Anatomy* and read it cover to cover.

People read inspiring words, listen to them at a seminar or on an instructional tape, and yet fail to act on the enthusiasm generated at the moment of impact. They slide back into their comfortable, if unhealthy, habits. This happens over and over again. I implore you not to be one of these people. Without knowing which vices you have (if any), I urge you to make a lifestyle change today. If any of the following applies to you, please understand that excessive drinking, smoking, drugs, junk food and a lazy attitude towards exercise are not to be part of your future. Regular workouts and wholesome, natural clean eating should be your new life. Follow my advice, pass it on to your family and offspring, get the word out and with any luck even those not yet born will one day benefit.

My greatest satisfaction has been in passing this healthful philosophy to generations of people like you who have read my books, listened to my seminars or watched me on TV. I want you

> **What is high on my list is the burning desire to help you improve your life.**

to embrace this new life with strength of purpose. I want you to keep it up for the rest of your happy, healthy long life. As I finish this book, I want you to remember: The most important person in the world is you. You came into this life alone and you're going to leave it alone. But in between, make the rest of your life the best of your life.

The rest of your life is the best of your life.

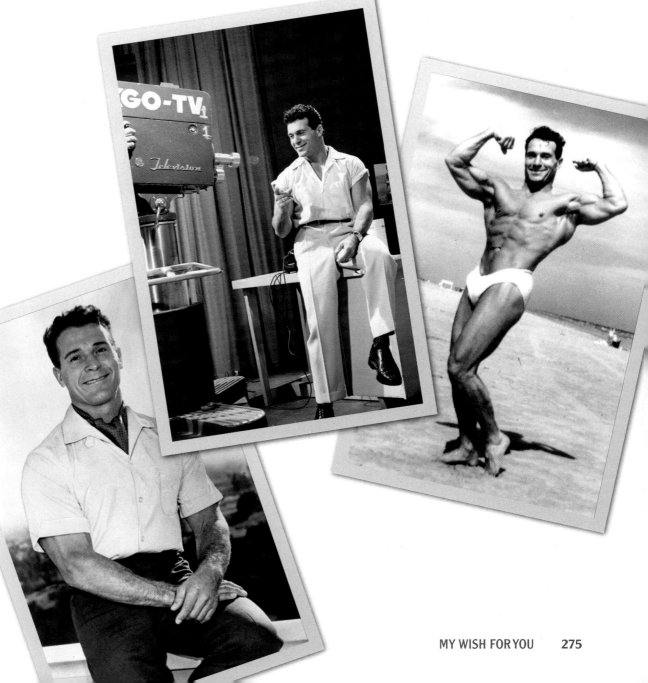

Jack La Lanne

ACHIEVEMENT TIMELINE

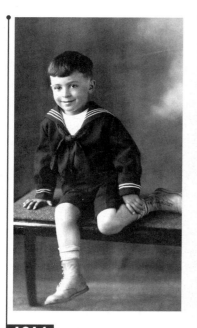

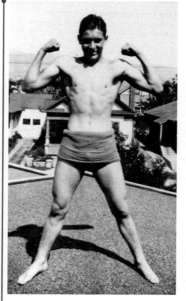

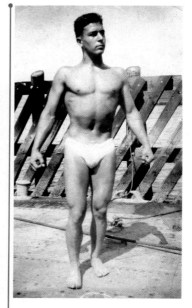

1914

I'm born in San Francisco, California on September 26. My journey has begun!

1930

At age 16, I've just discovered weight training and healthy nutrition. I'm on my way.

1932

I can hardly believe the progress I'm making with my health and physique. Now girls like me.

1914   1930   1932

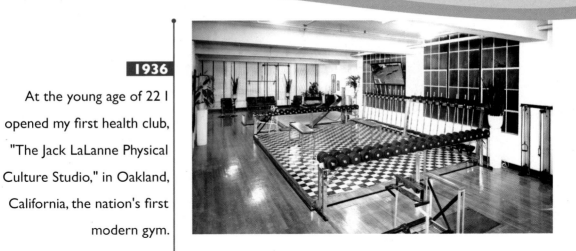

1936

At the young age of 22 I opened my first health club, "The Jack LaLanne Physical Culture Studio," in Oakland, California, the nation's first modern gym.

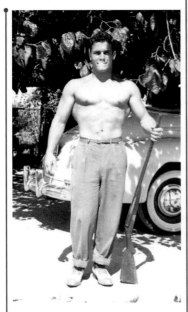

1935

I wanted to build a Mr. America-type body. And hey! The dream is becoming a reality.

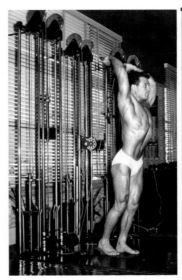

1936

I invented and pioneered the first selectorized weight apparatus and advanced pulley exercise machines, many of which are common in gyms today.

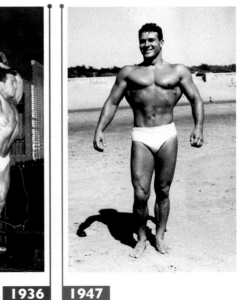

1947

I never gave up on my training and nutrition. At 33 my waist was still 27 inches, the same size as when I was 16.

1935   1936   1947

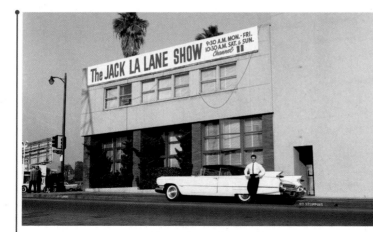

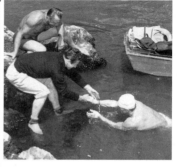

the **Jack LaLanne** show

1951

I began my TV program, *The Jack LaLanne Show*, which became the longest-running exercise show ever. Millions of people tuned in.

1954

I finally achieved my Mr. America-type physique, and it is showcased around the world on covers of fitness publications.

1955

For my 41st birthday I swam from Alcatraz Island to Fisherman's Wharf in San Francisco. (In cold, shark-infested waters, no less. Brrr.)

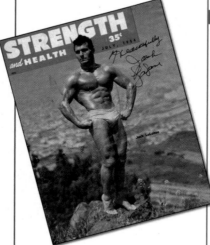

1951   1954   1955

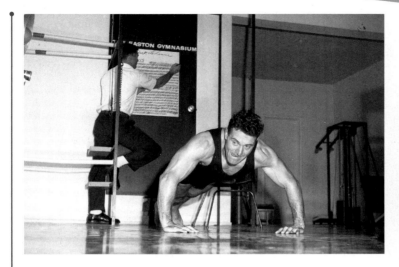

1956

I broke the world record by performing 1,033 pushups in 23 minutes on the popular TV show *You've Asked For It*, at age 42.

1957

To publicize my show and gym I towed a 2,500-pound, 19-foot Owens Cruiser through the Golden Gate Channel in San Francisco. The strong currents made the length of the swim equal 6.5 miles.

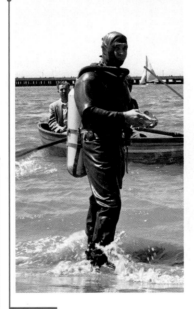

1961

At 47, I swam the entire length of the Golden Gate Bridge twice, underwater.

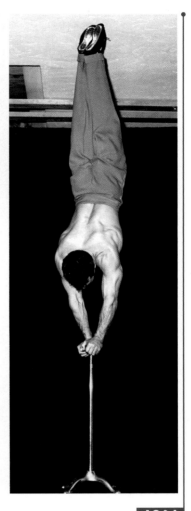

1964

At the age of 50 I headlined numerous stage and TV shows by performing an adagio (acrobalance) and hand-balancing act.

1956   1957   1961   1964

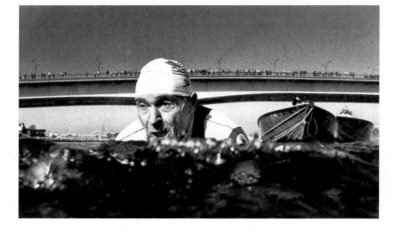

At age 70 I swam The Queen Mary Mile, towing 70 boats with one person in each boat for 1.5 miles, all against high winds and while handcuffed and shackled. This was probably my toughest feat.

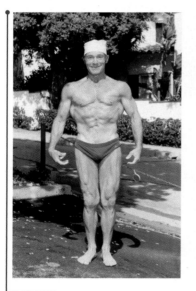

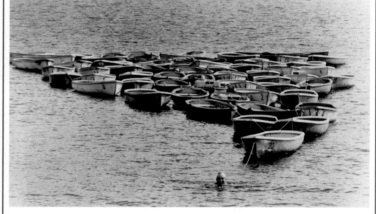

1979

On October 15, 1979 I swam Lake Oshinoko in Japan, again shackled and cuffed, pulling 65 boats loaded with 6,500 pounds of wood pulp (I'd just turned 65).

A year later in North Miami, Florida, I towed 10 boats filled with 77 people. I traveled one mile in under one hour.

1974

Shortly after my 60th birthday I swam (again) from Alcatraz Island to Fisherman's Wharf, but this time handcuffed and with my feet shackled.

1974   1979   1984

1994

I felt in top form at the age of 80, and I could still perform hundreds of non-stop pushups. I felt no different than I had at 25, a true testament to sensible exercise and nutrition. But the waistline was now 27 1/2 inches – up by half an inch. Ooops!

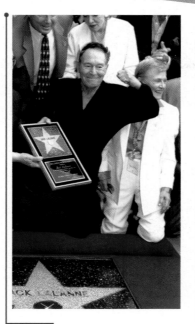

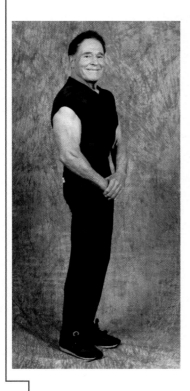

2002

On my 88th birthday I received my star on the "Hollywood Walk of Fame." At the same time I became the leading spokesperson for the Jack LaLanne Power Juicer, which has sold 1.8 million units worldwide.

2009

I wrote this book that you are now holding in your hands. At age 95 I love sharing my world with the joy of my life, Elaine. Our happiness has resulted from a commitment to loyalty, a common interest in keeping fit and healthy, and a fervent desire to help others.

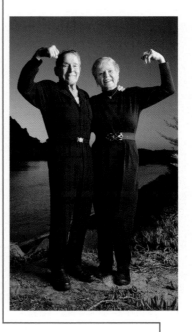

1994   2002   2009

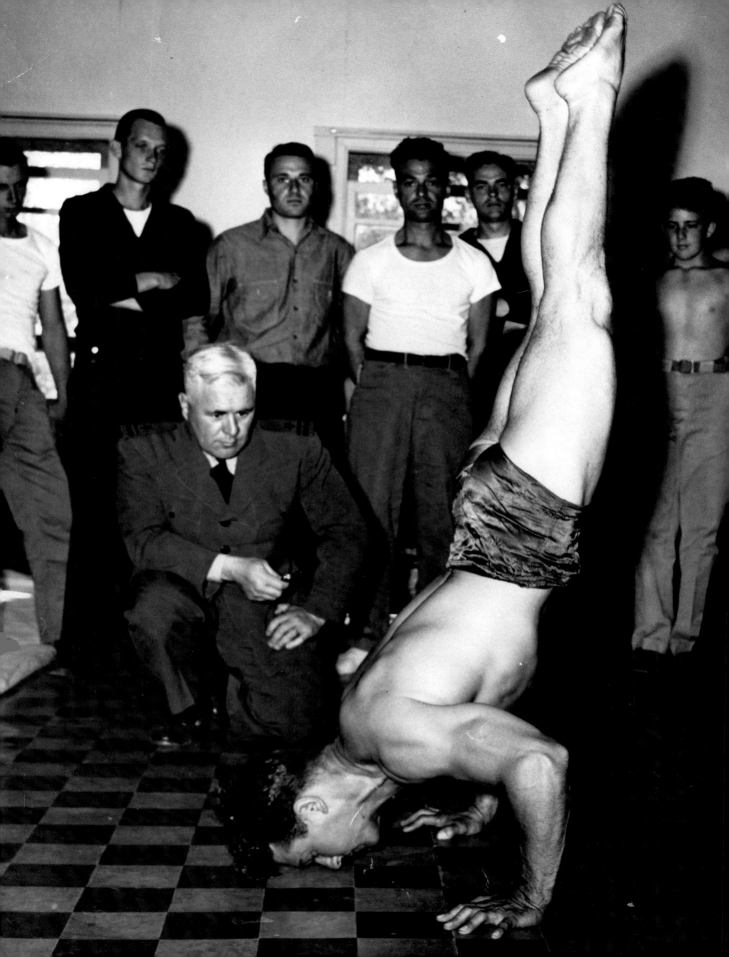

NMSH—FORM 33
(1939)

DO NOT ADDRESS THE SIGNER OF THIS LETTER
BUT ADDRESS YOUR REPLY TO
COMMANDING OFFICER
U. S. NAVAL HOSPITAL ________
AND REFER TO No.

U. S. NAVAL HOSPITAL

Sun Valley, Idaho

This is to certify that, Jack LaLanne, on the seventh day of August in the year 1944 performed 100 unsupported full hand stand press ups in the time period of five minutes and fifty seven seconds.

First witness and timekeeper for the event being Lt.(jg) Ralph A. Mazzei USNR.

Second witness and scorekeeper for the event being Joseph P. Stalego Phm.2/c USNR.

1st witness: Ralph A Mazzei
Ralph A. Mazzei
Lt.(jg) USNR
Physical Training Officer
U.S. Naval Convelescent Hospital
Sun Valley, Idaho

2nd witness: Joseph P Stalego PHM 2/c
Joseph P. Stalego Phm.2/c USNR
Physical Instructor

CREDITS

Brian Smith: Page 35, 49, 198, 272.

Fotolia.com: Page 267 (yams), 270 (bran).

iStockPhoto.com: Page 19-21, 25, 30-33, 37, 54, 63-69, 78, 84-85, 87, 91, 94, 97-98, 100, 104, 106, 112, 118-119, 121, 141-142, 144, 146, 150-151, 208-210, 212-213, 216-237, 244-271.

Paul Bucetta: Page 8.

Sandy DiPasquale: Page 130-134 (illustrations).

Ted Hammond: Page 135 (illustrations), 163-177 (illustrations), 180-197 (illustrations).

Vic Boff: Page 6.

INDEX

A

ABC-TV, 150
abdominals, 172-173, 190-191
acidity, 218
acting, 66, 201
adagio, 279
addiction, 64, 70
adrenal glands, 257
advice, 274-275
age, old, 44, 128
Agriculture Research Service, 221, 235
Alcatraz Island, 278, 280
alcohol, 67, 123, 141
alcoholics, 67
almonds, raw, 96
alpha-carotene, 259
Alzheimer's, 245, 260
American College of Sports Medicine, 126, 158
American Heart Association, 268
American Medical Association, 38
amino acids, 24, 232
anemia, 142, 230
anthocyanin, 235, 251
anti-aging, 222
anti-inflammatory, 245, 259, 262
antibiotic, 226
antioxidant, 217, 219-222, 226-227, 232, 234, 237, 249, 251, 256, 259-260, 262-263, 266, 268
apathy, 230
appearance, 76, 79, 113, 114, 119
apples, 217
approval, 72
apricots, 217, 218
ariels, 233
armpits, 76, 78
arms, 113
arteriosclerosis, 236
arthritis, 256, 262, 270
artichokes, 245
Ash, Carolyn, 81
asparagus, 245
asthma, 245, 256-257, 262, 266, 270
attractiveness, 112, 114
Australia, 36
auto accidents, 141
avocado, 213, 246

B

back, 24-25, 110, 112, 115, 134, 170-171, 188-189
back stretch, 134
bacteria, 122, 256, 269
bad breath, 38
Bakersfield, 18
baldness, 78
bananas, 213, 218
bank account, 32
Bank of Italy, 22
barley, 269
beans, 240
beating, 20
beets, 246
bell peppers, 258
Berkeley, California, 22, 25, 42
berries, 96, 103, 221
Bertinelli, Valerie, 206
beta-carotene, 217-218, 221, 227, 229, 234, 237, 248, 250, 262-264, 266-267
beta-cryptoxanthin, 229

beta-glucan fiber, 270
biceps, 176-177, 194-195
bioflavonoids, 223
birth defects, 245, 247, 249, 260
black currants, 219
blackberries, 220
blender, 213, 215
blood,
    clotting, 224, 226, 249, 254, 257, 262, 266
    drinking, 26
    pressure, 142, 234, 246, 253, 261, 264
    sugar regulation, 225, 229-231, 234, 256, 269, 270
blueberries, 221
body part, 160
bodybuilders, 126, 228
bodybuilding, 43
bodyfat, 121
bones, 156, 159, 217, 221, 225-227, 231-232, 237, 247, 249-251, 254, 257, 260, 266
born-again life, 23
bowel, 120, 229, 234, 257, 269
Bragg, Paul, 22-23, 90, 120, 274
bran, 269
BRAT diet, 218
Brazil nuts, 96
breads (including muffins and cakes), 96, 104, 241
breakfast, 103, 144
breast cancer, 221, 235, 247
brittle nails, 230
broccoli, 247
brown rice, 270
bruising, 223, 245
Brussels sprouts, 247
bulb, 267
Buying Fruits and Veggies, 96

C

cabbage, 248
caffeine, 123
caffeinated drinks, 123
calcium, 96, 247, 249, 257, 261-262, 264
calisthenics, 90
calories, 98, 105, 217, 218, 248, 249, 251, 254, 260
calves, 165, 182-183
Campoli, Dr. William, 85
cancer,
    breast, 221, 235, 247
    cervical, 221, 235, 265
    colon, 217, 223, 230, 234, 262, 264, 265, 270
    lung, 229
    preventing, 145, 217, 220, 222, 226, 233, 246-251, 259, 261-262, 265-267
    prostate, 258, 265
    rectal, 265
    skin, 81
canned foods, 98
cantaloupe melon, 221
carbohydrates, 144, 238, 263
cardiovascular disease, 217, 249, 255
cardiovascular system, 245, 264
career, 39
carotenoid, 229, 249
carrot, 248
cataracts, 247-249, 252
cauliflower, 249
cavities, 84
ceiling stretch, 130

celery, 249
cells, 100, 208, 232, 249, 259
cereal, 96-97, 144, 239
Charlotte, North Carolina, 85
chemicals, 90, 95, 210-212
cherries, 222
chest, 168-169, 192-193
chicken, 97
children, 36, 210, 248, 249
chiropractic degree, 30
cholesterol,
    controlling, 262, 270
    HDL (good), 222
    high, 55, 97, 253
    LDL (bad), 222, 224
    foods that lower, 217, 246, 261, 269
chromium, 256
Churchill, Winston, 156
cigar, 63
cigarettes, 55, 63-64, 79
circulation, 128-129, 142
circulatory conditions, 246
Cirque du Soleil, 127
cleanliness, 76
clogged pores, 78
cocoa butter, 82
coconuts, 213
coffee, 67, 68, 103, 215
Coffee and Alcohol Abuse, 67-68
colander, 215
collagen, 222, 231, 233, 247
collard greens, 250
colon, 120
    cancer, (see cancer)
    fiber, 231, 247, 269
coloring hair, 78
Commit Yourself, 62-63
confidence, 63, 128
constipation, 120, 217, 220, 230, 234, 251, 257
cooler, 98-99
coordination, 128
copper, 218, 234, 251, 269, 271
cotton products, 82
Countenance Counts, 110-115
crackers and crispbread, 242
cranberries, 222
creams, 82
crookneck, 262
cucumber, 250
Cyr, Diane, 10

D

Dad, 47-48
dairy, 242
dandruff, 78
dehydration, 121, 123, 147
Delmonteque, Dr. Bob, 110, 127
dementia, 245, 247, 249, 256
Dental Care, 84-85
dentist, 85
depression, 147, 230
dermatologists, 78
dessert, 103
diabetes, 217, 238, 268
digestion, 121, 218, 232
digestive tract, 215
Dining Out, 102-107

diseases, 66, 141
diuretic, 123, 245
diverticular disease, 223, 230, 251, 271
divorce, 153
dizziness, 230
doctors, 38
    approval, 158
    eye, 87
drinking problem, 55, 79
drug companies, 65
drug therapy, 65
drug use, 37-38
    recreational, 66
drugs, 65-66
DVD, 87

E

Eat A Balanced Breakfast, 144
economy, 36, 93
edema, 245
eggplant, 251
eggs, 97
ellagic acid, 221-222
Emotions: Anger And Fear, 143
energy, 39, 64, 143, 146, 208-209, 215, 218, 248, 251-252, 260
Everything Starts With A Thought, 36-39
excessive sunshine, 79
exercise, 13-14, 33, 42, 62
    effects of, 79, 156-157
    energy, 143
    eyes, 86-87
    intensity, 158-160
    lack of effects, 120
    motivation, 52-54
    starting, 158
    stress, 70
    stretching, 128
Extend Your Horizons, 126-128
Eye Care, 86-87
eyes, 63, 86-87, 147, 221, 225, 227, 237, 252, 258-260, 266
    puffiness, 250

F

face, 76
Facebook, 14
fast-food, 93
fat, 144, 158, 246, 260
fatigue, 140-147, 230, 264
Feeling Fresh, Healthy and Attractive, 76
fevers, 21
fiber, 120, 218, 220, 223, 226, 229-231, 234, 245-246, 251, 257, 259, 261, 263, 267, 269-271
figs, 223
fingertip pushups, 31
First Nations, 98
fish, 24, 97
Fisherman's Wharf, 278, 280
fizz, 118, 122
flavonoids, 220, 224, 233, 256
flexibility, 112, 126-128
flossing, 84
folate (folic acid), 96, 245, 247, 249, 251, 256-257, 260-261
food,
    box, 14, 93, 98
    can, 14, 97-98
    coloring, 209-210
    dinner party, 107
    farm grown, 90-91
    man-altered, 90, 93, 207
    nutritious, 99
    ordering at a restaurant, 103, 106
    prepackaged, 94
    price, 94
football, 25, 42, 102

Foreman, George, 206
fruit, 95, 216
    choosing, 96
    citrus, 214, 223
    dried, 218
    recommended servings, 210
    tropical, 225
    washing, 215
fungus, 255

G

gallbladder, 223, 250, 271
gardening, 145
gastrointestinal problems, 234
genus, 253
Get 20 Winks, 146
ginseng, 69
glands, 78, 217, 221, 225, 227, 237, 257
glutes, 184
Glycemic Index (GI) Food Chart, 239
Go Easy To Start, 158
goal, 110
goitrogens, 249
Golden Gate Bridge, 279
Golden Gate Channel, 279
government, 32
grains, 239, 268-271
grapefruit, 24, 223
grapes, 224-225
gravity, 113-114
gravy, 103
Gray's Anatomy, 23, 90, 274
Great Depression, 21-22
green beans, 251
green peas, 257
Greenfield, 18, 20
grocery shopping, 91, 94-95
    boxed products, 93
    farmers' markets, 93
    organically grown, 95
    produce, 91-93
groin, 76, 78
guavas, 225
Guide To Reducing Stress, 72-73
Gym Training, 180-197

H

HAAS, 246
hair, 221
    brushing, 78
    loss, 230
Hair Care, 78-79
hair dryer, 78
hair growth, 217
hairdressers, 78
hamstring stretch, 131
happiness, 76
headache, 20, 38, 230, 264
health, 36-37
hearing the message, 19-20
heart, 84, 218, 220, 224, 256
heart attack, 145, 230, 247, 262-263
heart disease, 222, 232-234, 247-248, 256, 259-260
hemorrhoids, 217, 220, 230, 234, 251, 257
hiking, 90
Hitler, 156
Hollywood Walk of Fame, 281
Home Training, 163-177
homocystein, 262-263
hoof-and-mouth disease, 22
hope, 23
Hopper, Hedda, 27
How To Begin Stretching, 129
How To Stay Motivated, 58
hydration, 118
hygiene, 76, 114

hypertension, 37, 260

I

ice packs, 99
iceberg lettuce, 254
ignorance, 95
immune system, 156, 217, 220, 227, 232, 236-237, 247, 257, 260, 271
indole-3-carbinol, 247-248
infection, 217, 219, 223, 227, 230, 237, 266
inflammation, 257
initiative, 32
injury, 42, 79, 126, 136, 159, 178
insulin, 144, 238
interest, 201
intestinal, 269
iron, 96-97
    deficiency, 230
    sources of, 226, 261, 264, 269
irritable bowel syndrome, 229-230, 261

J

Jack LaLanne
    Health Clubs, 105
    Physical Culture Studio, 277
    Power Juicer, 57, 102, 206, 281
    Special, 102
    Timeline, 276-281
jacked, 10
Japan, 280
Jenkins, Dr. David, 238
Jenny Craig, 206
Jesus, 10-11
Johns Hopkins Medical, 121
Johnson, Samuel, 37
joints, 127, 233, 256
juice, 24
    before meals, 215
    can or bottle, 208, 210
    coloring, 210
    fresh, 210
    storing, 214, 265
juicers, 206-207
juicing, 152, 206-207, 209-215, 235, 252
    avoid, 213
    weight loss, 209
    mangoes, 227
    seeds, 225
    skin on, 226, 231
    youth, 210
Juicing Tips, 214-215
jumping jacks, 10
junk food, 18-19, 38, 72, 79, 82

K

kale, 252
Keep Up With Your Workouts, 143
Kennedy, Robert, 45, 55
KGO-TV, 55, 150
kidney, 223, 246, 250, 261, 271
    stones, 222, 245
kiwi, 226
Kournikova, Anna, 206

L

Lake Oshinoko, 280
LaLanne, Elaine, 44, 102, 150-153, 207, 224, 281
lanolin, 82
laxative, 271
leeks, 213, 253
leg lunge stretch, 132
lemon, 226
lentil, 257
Let Me Take Your Hand, 30-34
lethargy, 145, 156
ligaments, 128, 250

limes, 227
Limit Your TV Time, 145
liver, 257
Long Beach Harbor, 10
longevity, 33, 76, 93
Lose The Scales, 158-159
lunch, 98, 146
lung cancer, 229
lycopene, 258, 265

M

magnesium, 218, 230, 256, 261, 264, 269, 271
manganese, 218, 220-221, 232, 234-236, 252-253,
    256-257, 261, 263-264, 269, 271
mangoes, 227
marital disharmony, 142
Markstein, Al, 43
martial arts, 42
Maximum Fitness, 45, 55
meat, 26, 97, 146
medical clinics, 95
Medical College of Wisconsin, 143
memory loss, 217
metabolism, 121, 156
military, 43
milk, 96, 242
minerals, 95, 122, 210, 212, 214, 230
mirror, 53, 62, 159
mobility, 112, 156
moderation, 25
Monday Night Football, 102
money, 38
mother, 18-19, 84
motivation, 52
    events, 57
    fear, 52
    mirror reflection, 53-54
    photos, 55, 58
    progress, 57
    reading, 55, 58
    romance, 52, 57
Mr. America, 43, 277
MuscleMag International, 45
muscles, 94, 126-128, 158-159, 229, 250, 264
Muscles Are Beautiful – and Useful, 156-157
mushrooms, 255
My Nutritional Passion: Juicing For Health, 206-212

N

naps, 146
nasunin, 251
National Aeronautics and Space Administration, 143
navy, 43
neck, 112
nectarines, 228
Nelson, Freddy, 47
nervous system, 236, 255-256
nervousness, 38, 70
neural-tube defects, 245
niacin, 234, 251, 269, 271
nicotine, 143
Nike, 206
nitrates, 122
nonorganic, 210, 212
North Miami, Florida, 280
nutrients, 207, 210, 214-215, 223, 237, 265, 268
nutritional intake, 32

O

Oakland, California, 9, 22, 26, 277
oatmeal, 103, 144, 270
obesity, 55, 147, 269
ocular lens, 257
odor,
    body, 76-77
    mouth, 84

oily skin, 82
okra, 256
onions, 256
optimist, 30, 42
oranges, 229
organic, 95, 210-212, 235
osteocalcin, 262, 264
osteoporosis, 128, 159, 224, 230
Other Causes Of Tiredness, 147
overstretching, 136
overweight, 82
oxalates, 223, 250
oxygen, 114, 121, 143, 264
Oxygen, 45, 55

P

pantothenic acid, 246, 251, 255
papain, 229
papaya, 229
Parkinson's disease, 245, 247, 249, 260
parsnips, 257
passion, 70
passion fruit, 230
pasta, 241
Paul Bragg seminar, 22, 90
peaches, 231
pears, 231
pelvis, 113
peptic ulcers, 248
periodontal disease, 85
perspiration glands, 78
pessimist, 30
pesticides, 95, 210
petroleum jelly, 82
phenols, 232
phosphorus, 96, 261, 269, 271
physical checkup, 62
physical fitness, 38
physical health, 53
physique, 256, 260
phytochemicals, 249
pilates, 72
pineapple, 232
pipe, 63
pith, 214
plan, 33, 72, 144
plaque, 84-85
plastic containers, 123
plums, 232
polyester, 82
pomegranate, 233
popsicle stick, 210
positive attitude, 58
posture, 110-115
    bad posture, 114-115, 147
    good posture, 114, 156
    lazy posture, 113
potassium, 96, 218, 220, 228-230, 234, 245-246, 251, 255,
    259, 261, 263-264, 267, 269-270
potatoes, 259
pregnant women, 123, 223, 249, 260
preparing, 70, 72
produce, 95, 210-212
proper nutrition, 52, 94
prostate cancer, 258, 265
protein, 24, 97, 144, 229, 247, 255, 261, 263-264, 269, 271
prunes (dried plums), 234
pulley exercise machines, 277
pumpkin, 259
pushups record, 279
psychological eater, 20

Q

quadriceps stretch, 134
Queen Mary Mile, 280
quercetin, 222, 235

Quinn, Dr. Tony, 111

R

radiation, 81
radicchio, 260
radishes, 260
ranch life, 18-19
range of motion, 126-128
raspberries, 235
realist, 30
rectal cancer, 265
relationship, 73, 152-153
relax, 72, 110-111
repetitions, 157, 160
Reps!, 45
resistance, 141
restaurants, 103-105
resveratrol, 224
retirement, 200-202
rhubarb, 213
riboflavin, 96, 251, 255, 269
Rolex, 206
romaine lettuce, 254
Russian River, 47

S

salad, 13, 97, 103, 105
Salt Lake, 24
San Francisco, 48, 90, 150, 202, 276, 278-279
Santa Monica, 86
Say No To Tobacco, 143
scales, 158
scalp oil, 78
Schwarz, Harry, 105
scientific progress, 36
scurvy, 227
seated hamstring stretch, 133
sebaceous glands, 78
selectorized weight apparatus, 277
selenium, 96, 269-271
self esteem, 54
server, 103, 104-107
Seventh Day Adventist, 21
sex appeal, 114
sex drive, 128, 153
sexual activity, 142, 147
shampoo, 78
Sheridan, Dr. David, 144
shoulder stretch, 133
shoulders, 113, 133, 166-167, 185-187
Showering, 76-78
side-to-side stretch, 130
silica, 250
Simmons, Richard, 45
skin, 79-82
    cancer, 81
    clear, 219
    eruptions, 38
    healthy, 217, 221-222, 225, 227, 231-232, 237, 250, 255,
        259, 266
    problems, 79
    water, 119
Skin Care, 79-81
sleep,
    enhancer, 222
    lack of, 79, 113, 140-141
Smoking, 63-64
    effects of, 79, 143
smoothies, 215, 218
snacks, 242
soap, deodorant, 78
sodium, 122
soy, 97, 261
soybeans, 261
Spain, 265
speeches, 70

spina bifida, 245
spinach, 262
Splash Publishing, 81
squash, 262
stamina, 24, 126, 230
standing calf stretch, 135
stiffness, 126
stimulant, 68, 143
stomach, 68, 110, 218
straight neck, 262
strawberries, 236
stress, 69-73
    control, 112
    effects of lifestyle, 79
    overcoming, 70-73
stress test, 62, 158
Stressed Out, 69-70
stretching, 126-136
Stretching Principles, 136
stroke, 52, 230, 233, 246-247, 253, 257, 261-263, 268, 270
sugar, 18, 207
sugarholic, 31, 207
sunbathing, 147
sunburn, 250
sunflower seeds, 96
sunshine, 79-81
    protection, 81
sweating, 78-79
sweet potato, 263
swelling, 245
Swiss chard, 264

T
Tackle One Thing At A Time, 144
Take A Vacation, 146
Taking On Extra Activities, 145
tan, 79
tanning beds, 81
tannins, 224, 235
tartar, 84
teenage years, 24
teeth, 84-85, 225, 227
tendons, 128, 159
The Fatigue Factor, 140-142
The Jack Lalanne Show, 53, 278
The Physician and Sports Medicine, 159
thiamin, 251, 261, 269, 271
Thighs, 163-164, 180-181
through the legs stretch, 131
thyroid,
    normal function, 232
    problems, 249
    underactive, 142
tiger stretch, 132
Timeless Skin, 81
Tips On Keeping Your Skin Healthy and Looking Good, 82
tiredness, 140-141, 144-145, 156-157
tissues, 79, 143, 257
tobacco, 63, 143
toe touch, 135
tofu, 97
tomatoes, 265
Tomorrow Is What You Eat Today, 90-95
tooth decay, 222
toothbrush, 84-85
tough love, 54-55
toxins, 121, 213
training, 129, 143, 159
    frequency, 160
    men compared to women, 178
travel, 99, 145
Travel Can Be Exhausting, 145
treadmill, 72, 129
triceps, 174-175, 196-197
tropical vine, 267

turnips, 266
TV, 145
Twitter, 15
Two Are Better Than One, 150-153

U
uncontrollable rages, 20
unhealthiness, 66
University of South Carolina, 144
University of Toronto, 238
urinary calcium excretion, 245
urinary tract infection, 222, 224
USDA, 210, 244

V
vacation, 146
vegetables, 95, 97, 212, 244-267
    choosing, 96
    juicing, 206, 210, 214-215
    leafy, 264
    root, 266
vegetarian, 21, 23
    protein, 97
visualize, 58
vitamins, 69, 95, 145, 212, 214, 237
vitamin A, 221, 227, 237, 248, 249, 250, 254, 259, 263, 264, 266, 267
    excellent sources of, 217-218, 221, 223, 227, 230, 234, 248, 250, 252-254, 256-257, 259, 262-266
vitamin B6, 259, 262-263
    excellent sources of, 218, 234, 259, 263, 267, 269, 271
vitamin C, 219, 220, 221, 223, 225, 226, 227, 232, 233, 236, 247, 249, 250, 256, 257, 260, 262, 266
    deficiency, 231, 245
    excellent sources of, 217, 219-227, 229-230, 232, 235-237, 245-248, 250-252, 256-267
vitamin E, 96, 232
    excellent sources of, 250
vitamin K, 226, 249, 250, 254, 257, 262, 264, 266
    excellent sources of, 221, 224, 226, 245-248, 250-254, 257, 262, 264, 266

W
walking, 42, 72, 150
warm up, 126, 129
watcher of people, 34
water, 99, 118-123
    body usage, 120
    breathing, 121
    cold, 123
    dehydration, 123
    distilled, 122
    filter, 122
    iceberg lettuce, 254
    mineral, 122
    older people, 119
    pregnant, 123
    table, 123
    unfiltered tap, 119
    vegetables, 120
Water Drinking, the Do's and Don'ts of, 122-123
water-soluble, 219-220, 225, 232, 236, 250, 257, 267
watercress, 266
watermelon, 237
weakness, 230-231
wealth, 38-39
weight training, 57, 157, 159-160, 276
weights, 25
Weights Are Great, 159
wellness factor, 38
We're Only Human, 42-48
wheat, 271
white blood cells, 219, 221, 227
white rice, 270
wild mushrooms, 255
willpower, 58

Women's City Club, 22
Woods, Tiger, 206
work, 200
work out, 72, 156-160
World War II, 43, 156
wound healing, 219, 221, 227, 266
wrestling, 25, 274
writing, 201

Y
yams, 267
YMCA, 25, 274
yoga, 72
You've Asked For It, 279
Young, Dr. Vicky, 143
Your Body Is Thirsting For Water., 118-123
Your Essential Starting Point., 52-57
Your Home Training Routine, 162
youth, 18-22

Z
zinc, 96, 269, 271
zucchini, 120, 262